100 Questions & Answers About Schizophrenia: Painful Minds

THIRD EDITION

Lynn Eleanor DeLisi, MD

JONES & BARTLETT
LEARNING

World Headquarters
Jones & Bartlett Learning
5 Wall Street
Burlington, MA 01803
978-443-5000
info@jblearning.com
www.jblearning.com

Jones & Bartlett Learning books and products are available through most bookstores and online booksellers. To contact Jones & Bartlett Learning directly, call 800-832-0034, fax 978-443-8000, or visit our website, www.jblearning.com.

Substantial discounts on bulk quantities of Jones & Bartlett Learning publications are available to corporations, professional associations, and other qualified organizations. For details and specific discount information, contact the special sales department at Jones & Bartlett Learning via the above contact information or send an email to specialsales@jblearning.com.

Production Credits
Executive Editor: Nancy Anastasi Duffy
Editorial Assistant: Jade Freeman
Production Manager: Daniel Stone
Production Services Manager: Colleen Lamy
Marketing Manager: Lindsay White
Manufacturing and Inventory Control Supervisor: Amy Bacus
Composition: Miranda Design Studio, Inc.
Cover Design: Stephanie Torta
Rights & Media Research Assistant: Wes DeShano
Media Development Editor: Shannon Sheehan
Cover Image: Top Left: © AbleStock; Top Right: © Photodisc; Bottom Left: © Photos.com; Bottom Right: Purestock/Thinkstock
Printing and Binding: Edwards Brothers Malloy
Cover Printing: Edwards Brothers Malloy

Library of Congress Cataloging-in-Publication Data
DeLisi, Lynn E.
100 questions and answers about schizophrenia : painful mind / Lynn DeLisi. — Third edition.
pages cm
Includes bibliographical references and index.
ISBN 978-1-284-06576-3 (alk. paper)
1. Schizophrenia—Popular works. I. Title. II. Title: 100 questions and answers about schizophrenia. III. Title: One hundred questions & answers about schizophrenia.
RC514.D45 2016
616.89'8—dc23
2015024007

978-1-284-06576-3

6048

Printed in the United States of America
19 18 17 16 10 9 8 7 6 5 4 3 2 1

Dedication

This edition is dedicated to all families worldwide who suffer because they have one or more relatives with schizophrenia; to those individuals whose goals for life have been destroyed by this illness; and to those professionals who have devoted their lives to the service of patients with serious mental illness.

CONTENTS

Part 2: Treatment: When, Where, by Whom, and With What? *53*

Questions 25–41 review different options available to treat schizophrenia:

Part 3: Genetic Risk *91*

Questions 42–57 discuss the genetic risks associated with schizophrenia:

Part 4: Nongenetic Risk Factors *121*

Questions 58–64 discuss nongenetic-based risk factors that can contribute to schizophrenia:

ACKNOWLEDGMENT

The author would like to acknowledge the Staglin family, founders of the IMHRO/One Mind Institute, for what they are doing to make progress toward the understanding of schizophrenia.

Psychiatric illnesses are the number one cause of disability worldwide. The global economic burden from mental illnesses is estimated at nearly $2.5 trillion dollars annually. Over 1 million people each year will end their lives in suicide, and about 90% of these people will have had a psychiatric condition. IMHRO is an organization established to facilitate effective approaches for recovery for persons with mental illness, and even cures. It was founded in 1995 by Shari and Garen Staglin, who, inspired by their experience with their son Brandon's schizophrenia diagnosis and recovery, realized that "running toward the problem" could provide solutions not just for their own family, but for people everywhere affected by mental illness. Since then, their tireless work, with their board and staff, has transformed the landscape of brain health research and inspired advocates around the world. They provide funds to promising neuroscientists who are growing our knowledge of psychiatric disease and developing exciting new treatments. The proceeds from the sale of this book will be donated to IMHRO in support of their effort.

In addition, the author would like to acknowledge all the patients and families with schizophrenia who have contributed to her understanding of this disorder.

A Patient's Perspective

As I know first-hand, schizophrenia is a terrifying, sometimes unbearably painful and mysterious affliction. Many non-afflicted people fear schizophrenia, and fear individuals who live with the disease. This fear is deepened by the fact that many know so little about schizophrenia's causes, symptoms, and prognosis. Even I, a person who has lived with the disease since 1990, knew little about it until about 15 years after I was diagnosed. As science and treatment progress, I am still learning, and books such as *100 Questions & Answers About Schizophrenia* are helping me to deal with it better, for what it is.

My personal journey with schizophrenia began in my teenage years, when early warning signs began to appear. Around age 16, I began to spend most of my free time by myself, taking long hikes and bike rides through the countryside around my home and school. My thoughts on these forays strayed increasingly into mystical ideas, contemplating, for example, how "cool" it would be if spirits lived in the trees in a valley below, or how spooky that unfamiliar, shadowy trail looked. The academic and social stress of my first year of college probably compounded my disease's progression, for the following summer I withdrew further: I stopped reading and playing computer games, two of my favorite hobbies up to that time. I heard mocking voices in my head call me "Baby Brandon" and "Mixed Up Kid." I began to behave erratically; for example, I took a two-hour detour on what would have been a half-hour late-night drive because I felt I could not bear the predictability of my life.

One night that summer, a psychotic break stripped me of my sense of identity, and of the "correctness" of my experience of the world. From that moment when I felt the tension in my face "snap" and my emotions swirl into giddy unrecognizability, all calm, all joy, and all love I could remember feeling were gone. What I recall most clearly about the arduous months that followed were the moment-to-moment steps I took to avoid my worst fear: that the slightest mistake would literally send me to hell for all eternity. I covered my right eye, so a malevolent spirit would not enter there and take over my body. I avoided eating too many bites of lunch, as I "knew" that too much food would mean I would go to hell instantly. I clenched my toes, so my soul would stop leaking out of my feet. Every day felt like survival. One day, I was so sure I would fail that I came close to deciding to end it all myself.

And still, I could not accept that I was mentally ill. "Crazy," in my mind, was the worst thing you could call someone. I vehemently denied that I was sick, and railed against taking the medication I had been prescribed. Despite my parents' prohibition and my sister's protests, I sneaked out of my house to drive my car, when even I subconsciously knew I could not drive safely. My relationship with my parents grew strained. As hard as my disease was for me, I know now that it was very hard for them, too.

But, God bless them, they would not give up on me, and thanks in part to their persistence, I did not give up either. When my Dad told me one miserable afternoon, "There's a lot of love coming from here, Brandon," somehow it reached me. In that moment I knew I wanted to be able to return that love again someday. I took my medication thereafter, volunteered as a primate research assistant at the Oakland Zoo, and began to audit classes at UC Berkeley. The treatment and community involvement worked. By December, I had recovered well enough to go back to college, and to ultimately succeed there. Today, I am working, married, own a wonderful dog, and live a life filled with meaning.

My parents started their nonprofit, IMHRO, which funds brain disease research, in 1995. Working with it since 2005, I have learned a lot about what psychiatric disease is, and about the hope implicit in current cutting-edge research. As IMHRO's Communications Director, I have learned so much from my contact with many families and individuals with schizophrenia.

Even after decades of brain research, so many are still suffering so deeply. This suffering, due to the symptoms, the stigma, the perceived hopelessness, and the current dysfunction of much of our nation's mental health care system, is still compounded by the mystery surrounding schizophrenia. Many families and individuals want to know: What warning signs should I look for? What treatments and approaches can help? Why did our loved one get schizophrenia? Does the disease potentially limit his or her life prospects? Is there hope for a better life? In this book, Dr. DeLisi's comprehensive, no-nonsense coverage of the facts and statistics give an authoritative and compassionate perspective on this disease.

The more people understand about schizophrenia, the less they will irrationally fear it, and the better equipped they will be to deal with it. I hope that the power in this knowledge will encourage more people to speak openly about schizophrenia in their own lives, and to actively support the research and policy advances which will be necessary to ensure better recovery prospects for the millions suffering. In this regard, *100 Questions & Answers About Schizophrenia* offers useful knowledge. I hope that reading this book will benefit you as it has benefited me.

Brandon Staglin
Rutherford, California
October 3, 2014

A Sister's Perspective

Many remarkable individuals have suffered from schizophrenia, such as my brother, Scott David Shannon, a man of incredible courage, compassion, and intelligence. Growing up as his twin sister, I knew him well. Some of my first memories are of laughing with him while our young Mom pushed us down the slightly sloping and bumpy village sidewalk of Shirley Street in Shortsville, New York in a double stroller. Scott and I held hands on our first day of kindergarten, were read to in our pajamas on either side of Mom while in bed, ran with other kids in the "pickle-shaped" park in the middle of our street during the afternoons, and often played Monopoly and other board games inside on rainy days. We had an easy middle-class life despite our father living separately in Maryland and only rarely calling, visiting, or providing any type of support. Scott and I had a stable and loving home with our mother, Carol Ann, and grandfather, Elger, both working full-time, while our stay-at-home grandmother, Alice, did the cooking and cleaning. I remember that when our grandmother was making a yummy cake for dinner, she would offer Scott and me one of the electric mixer whisks to lick when we got home from school. Grandma Alice made sure we went to Sunday school and church. Our family life was not exactly tranquil, however, with often heated conversations over political and social issues argued over the dinner table or in the family living room.

In elementary school, Scott and I both found that good grades came to us easily, although like most children, we had to be told to do our homework. We both looked forward to summertime with swimming in the neighbor's pools, the days at the Roseland amusement park, weeklong vacations at the 4-H Camp Bristol Hills, and trips to the cabin on Blue Mountain Lake in the Adirondacks with our grandparents. In the mountains, Scott would go boating and fishing with Grandpa, and I would pick black-eyed Susan flowers and drink hot tea with Grandma. Once, Scott and I raced up Blue Mountain for about an hour, and Scott emerged victorious, arriving at the summit first. We stayed on top of the mountain just long enough to see the view with the expanse of evergreen trees and shimmering lake below, but we could not wait to race back down—and I arrived at the bottom ahead of Scott! We were generally in competition with each other in academics as well; for example, in high school we both worked towards the best grade in algebra, which our Grandfather forewarned us would be a "tough" subject. That year, Scott was only 2 points behind my score of 100 on the state-wide Regents Exam in algebra, and one year later, I was 2 points behind his score of a 98 in geometry. We both loved math and found the academic aspects of high school a lot less challenging than the social aspect. We were both physically small and not very athletic, and consequently we were often the last chosen for athletic teams, which did not help our self-esteem. I remember feeling awkward at my first teenage party, not knowing where to stand or who to talk to and being glad when it was over. When I was about 15 or 16, some neighborhood boys started hanging around my house and my best friends' house. I remember that my brother would stand on the front porch yelling at those boys to get off the lawn, and I thought, "Why was he acting that way?"

My whole family (Grandpa, Grandma, and Mom) all smoked cigarettes, and so it was no surprise that Scott and I both tried cigarettes when we were teens. Scott got hooked on smoking at around 16 years of age. He had a neighborhood best friend, Doug, who would accompany him everywhere. Scott liked to speed on his Yamaha motorcycle on dirt paths with Doug holding on for his life. We all listened to rock music in the early 1980s and Scott idolized Jim Morrison of The Doors.

It was around this time that I started to notice a big change in my brother. Normally, our school made an effort to separate twins into different sections, and trigonometry was the first class that Scott and I had together. When I found myself becoming confused, I remember glancing over at Scott, and instead of seeing him concentrating on the lecture and taking notes, I noticed that his eyes were glazed over and he was often staring out the window.

I thought to myself, "What was he doing?" He clearly was not paying attention to the teacher during class, but instead he seemed to have been starting to withdraw and descend into a scary and strange new world.

I also began to realize that something was wrong with Scott after waking up one night and hearing him crying to my mother about how he felt bullied in school and that he had no friends. I could certainly relate to his feelings, since I also found high school to be a difficult time for me. My Mom thought that a change of scene would solve our problems, so Scott, my Mom, and I all moved to a new town and I started a new high school, and my brother took his high school courses at a community college. My Mom helped Scott buy his first car so he could drive to college. Mom also helped Scott obtain a summer job with the engineering department at Mobil Chemical where she worked, while I worked at McDonald's serving Big Macs and fries with a friendly smile. My brother was so excited, and at first loved the change; he excelled in the company of scientists and was considered a "boy genius," writing computer programs that helped regulate shipments out of the plant. Scott felt like he had found his ideal job working with the engineering department, since he loved math and science, and he imagined himself as an engineer someday working in a laboratory.

All of my brother's dreams came to a screeching halt when he lost control of his thoughts and feelings. I remember one day hearing the familiar Doors music coming from his bedroom, so I thought that I would go in to listen and spend some time with him. I knocked and received no response. I opened the door only to find all kinds of hand-colored paper pyramids and triangles strategically positioned around the room, some on top of his record turnstile, and clothing hangers that were bent into antenna shapes. I remember thinking, "Wow, this is all very strange." But it was not strange to Scott. To him there was a perfectly reasonable explanation for it all: This arrangement was designed by Scott to enable him to receive special messages that were meant only for him. Of course, this made the whole situation appear even weirder to me.

I also remember sharing our birthday cake when we turned 17 years old, and I thought that everything was okay until Scott announced to our Mom and grandparents that I was the daughter of the devil. We all thought that surely Scott was not serious, and that he was saying things to get a reaction from us, but he continued to insist; he explained that he knew of the very dark and evil things that were occurring in the world, and his sentences would lose meaning as he fused one paranoid and bizarre thought into another. As Scott's 17-year-old twin, his behavior frightened me. I did not understand it, and I found myself not wanting to stay at home. I found every excuse to go out in the evening. This left my Mom at home to try to help Scott think clearly and to see reality. Unfortunately, this approach did not work, and my brother turned on our Mom one night; he hurt her physically by knocking her against a wall, and he threatened to harm her more. I was at home that night when my Mom screamed for me to help and call the police. It was horrific to see the police take my twin brother away from home, but it was the only thing my Mom and I could do. Mom went to the police station, but my brother was so psychotic that he claimed she was not his mother; in his "reality," Yoko Ono was his mother. He said many other things that did not make sense, and the police recognized that my brother seriously needed a psychiatric evaluation.

At that time, during the early 1980s, my brother was placed in a large state psychiatric hospital. He looked much like a scared young boy among a ward full of older people, some of whom were pacing, drooling, or rocking back and forth and appearing only so very ill. It was a terrible shock to see him in a stark white room, and even worse to see him struggle with medication. He was placed on a high dose of what are now called first-generation antipsychotic medications that made him feel very uncomfortable. My mom and

I later discovered that his experience with antipsychotic medicine was the most horrible experience of his life; Scott explained that he would rather die than have to go through this experience at the psychiatric ward again. When he returned home to live with my grandparents, I remember that he would pace the floor, and eventually he developed tardive dyskinesia, which is uncontrollable movements of the mouth. Seeing my twin brother suffer with his illness and the horrible side effects of his inadequate treatment motivated me to dedicate my life to research the underlying cause of this devastating disorder, and to develop better and more rational treatments. I knew that I wanted to try to understand the brain on the cellular and molecular level, but I did not even know the field of neuroscience existed when I made this commitment after high school. So I studied both biology and psychology in college, went on to graduate school, and then later postdoctoral training, eventually establishing my own research laboratory.

In the late 1980s, the most prominent theory of schizophrenia centered on the dopamine system, but I had always viewed schizophrenia as a developmental disorder, since I had grown up with a "normal" twin brother who eventually changed into someone I could not recognize during our adolescent years. I experienced similar biological changes and social challenges as a teenager as Scott did, but Scott's life took a dramatically different course. I wanted to understand if the typical changes that occur during brain maturation did not occur properly in the brains of people who suffered from schizophrenia, especially as I began to realize that my brother's story was common. Many people who develop schizophrenia first experience their symptoms during late adolescence or early adulthood after a relatively normal childhood.

So my quest to understand schizophrenia and develop better treatments was born in the living room of my childhood home in the early 1980s. By the time I had my own research program on schizophrenia, my brother was receiving the newer second-generation antipsychotic medication; Scott finally appeared to improve and he began feeling much better. However, he still spent the majority of his time in his bedroom, studying math and science books or reading novels. He did manage to get out of our childhood home and helped elderly neighbors by bringing them to their doctor appointments, shoveling snow from their sidewalks, and delivering "meals on wheels." He even traveled to England with me and my husband. Scott was able to tour a country he had only dreamed of visiting. He also attended photography classes at the community college and chemistry classes taught by some of my former teachers at Keuka College with the hope of assisting me in my research laboratory some day. Although he felt the social stress of the classroom interfered with his learning and test taking, he was able to complete three semesters. I bought a house where Scott intended to come to live with me some day. Although Scott was improved psychologically from the newer medication, he had excessive weight gain and suffered from diabetes, which can be a common side effect of antipsychotic medication.

I was recruited to Sydney, Australia to lead a schizophrenia research program, and although it was far away from my brother, I had an opportunity to double my research team, develop a department, and lead research focused on the developmental neurobiology of schizophrenia. We also hope to make progress toward developing new medications that will further improve the lives of people with schizophrenia. Although my twin brother, Scott, prematurely passed away a few years ago, I hope that one day we will have answers to prevent and cure this terrible disease so that other people will not suffer as he did.

A diagnosis of a disease such as schizophrenia, often thought to be "all in your mind," leaves patients and their loved ones filled with questions and fears. This makes a book such as *100 Questions & Answers About Schizophrenia* very important. Dr. DeLisi's book fills the need for comprehending a misunderstood illness such as schizophrenia. Using this book as a resource will provide the knowledge that is necessary to cope with the diagnosis of mental illness. The psychic pain of mental illness is often as hard to bear as the physical pain of a cancer. However, there is hope for a positive outcome in the future made possible by continuing research such as that done by Dr. DeLisi, myself, and our colleagues.

Cyndi Shannon-Weickert, PhD
Sydney, Australia

*The Nurses' Perspective**

I turned my head away, embarrassed for the stranger I did not even know. I started to talk to my husband because I did not want him to see the person walking on the sidewalk. The man had many layers of clothing on and was filthy. He appeared to be having a whole conversation with himself, and, by the appearance of things he had in a shopping cart along side of him, must have been homeless. As a young child, my mother had told me to stay away from "those people" because they were "crazy" and may hurt me.

One night, after turning my head away from "those crazy" people for several years, my whole life and understanding changed. I started a job working the night shift on a 28-bed admitting psychiatric unit, and it was time to face my fears. As I locked the door behind me, I wondered if this was something I was capable of doing, if I would ever stop being afraid. Twenty years later, I am still caring for this population as a Registered Nurse, and I can't imagine doing anything else. I am no longer afraid and now can see that I was afraid because I did not understand mental illness.

Working on an admitting psychiatric unit has allowed me to know some of the most acutely and severely ill individuals. Helping these patients to gain as much independence as they are capable of, remain in the community, think about recovering, and meanwhile manage the illness and its symptoms, are all important aspects of my job.

*Disclaimer: The views expressed in this foreword are those of the authors and do not reflect the official policy of The Department of the Army, Department of Defense, Veteran Affairs, or the U.S. Government.

The hardest part of my role, however, is fighting the stigma attached to this mental illness. Sadly, while it is the illness that causes the stigma, it is the *person* who is stigmatized. With no understanding of the illness, many people are afraid of a person who has schizophrenia. The portrayal of the illness on television and in the news media supports this fear and increases the stigma.

I have now been teaching the new nurses who will care for these patients in the future. I teach mental health nursing to student nurses during their mental health rotation and also new graduate nurses assigned to my service. The first day is always the same: They enter the inpatient setting with looks of fright on their faces, and while they all say they are not afraid to enter a locked psychiatric unit, it is obvious by their faces how frightened they really are. They come to the unit with a preconceived notion of what they will encounter. Many have said that they expected to be entering a very violent environment and that the patients would be delusional or yelling and screaming.

Patients with schizophrenia are the ones that students and new nurses seem to fear the most, and this fear appears to be based on the stigma associated with mental illness and the lack of education specifically about this illness in school. New nurses and students have not experienced knowing people with schizophrenia and thus lack the ability to fully comprehend their pain, having only read about the illness in their textbooks, some of which contain outdated information. They are also fearful because they do not understand how a person can hear voices or see things that are not really there. They wonder how they will ever understand what is occurring in the mind of such a patient, and struggle with providing care for an illness they cannot see.

Newly graduated registered nurses Kelly Coughlan, BSN, and Kathleen Nguyen, BSN, shared with me their thoughts and feelings they remember having during their first days assigned to a psychiatric unit and caring for patients with schizophrenia:

What is my role? What is a a psychiatric nurse supposed to do? Will it be scary? Could I get hurt? Question after question flooded my brain as I anticipated the start of my first job as a registered nurse. My experience working with the mentally ill was limited. The negative stigma surrounding these patients only added to my anxiety toward beginning this new experience, and I had no idea what to expect.

The patients I encountered with a diagnosis of schizophrenia were the scariest to me. I observed that some were angry, some appeared disheveled, and some were laughing hysterically to themselves, while others appeared "normal" until they began spewing non-sense that I could hardly decipher. The most unsettling part for me was that I didn't know what to expect from any one of them.

Some of the patients displayed odd and inappropriate behaviors that made me uncomfortable. I was confused about how to handle the strange behaviors we witnessed daily. What I learned quickly was that no two patients behave the same way, and they each have their own unique personalities just like any other human being and that part is not "illness", but what a nurse in any specialty learns to enjoy in this caring profession.

Initially, caring for patients with schizophrenia did not seem rewarding, as I was saddened to see them struggle to find and keep housing, and frustrated when they refused the medications I knew they desperately needed. Their delusions and paranoia inhibited me from communicating with each patient in the way I had in nursing school with patients who had other medical illness. It was difficult to speak their language and unsatisfing not to. Over time, I began to learn new methods of communication. Often, the techniques needed to successfully communicate with patients are as basic as being a good listener and having the patience and time to listen. Simply being present, acknowledging the patient's reasoning may be enough to earn their trust. Although their thoughts may be irrational or lack insight, their concerns deserve to be heard and the caregivers need to be respectful of the patients' feelings and fears no matter how delusional they may be, doing one's best to put the patients at ease.

I have learned that the ability to earn a patient's trust is the most important tool to deliver the best care that they deserve. Hopefully, I have a long nursing career ahead of me, and I'll take the skills I have learned working with schizophrenia patients and apply them to communicate and care for all of my future patients. This unique population continuously teaches me about myself and the kind of nurse that I hope to become, and I am wholeheartedly grateful for the opportunity.

Kelly A. Coughlan, BSN, RN

When I first heard that I was going to be working on an acute psychiatry unit, I was excited about my first job, but nervous about the unknown challenges of working in such a unique field. It didn't take long before I found myself interested in learning about schizophrenia and what that illness entailed. It only took a couple days to realize how flawed my initial perceptions had been. I came with the idea that people with schizophrenia always look disheveled, murmur to themselves while responding to auditory hallucinations, as well as act bizarre and have an inability to communicate. My biggest concern was that I would not be able to understand them and their actions would be unpredictable. Since working on this unit, I have found that people with schizophrenia vary considerably. There are some patients who need constant redirection, those who are responding to voices and those who appear detached; but most importantly, these patients are not causing harm to others and are respectable and friendly despite their illnesses. Many people identify schizophrenia as something that characterizes those we hear about on the news who have committed a terrible, violent act; the patients who are released from hospitals, act in a state of violence, claim insanity, and are eventually placed in state forensic mental institutions. As a society, we are quick to accept these instances as the norm, or even stereotypes, but because we keep hearing these cases in the news we forget that violence is rarely a characteristic of the illness. Many of the patients have no violent history and would never consider acting out such behavior. In fact, many patients have stated that they would rather harm themselves before harming anyone else.

I have cared for many patients now and have noticed some similarities and differences between them. The resounding similarity among these patients is the constant struggle of fitting into the social norm or society's perception of a "normal" individual. I have realized that a patient with schizophrenia does have the ability to maintain functionality if permitted within society. A common misperception among patients is the idea that once they are stable and are functioning properly, they no longer need the assistance of their medications. These are the times where their symptoms slowly begin to creep up, families become wary about their loved ones, and professional help is required once again. There are many patients who succumb to substance abuse and homelessness, yet many are functional with steady jobs, families and seemingly normal lives. I have witnessed the mannerisms of a patient and how we are quick to stare and assume "psychosis," which leads most of us to avoid them because it makes their differences uncomfortable to us. It is intensely apparent how, over time, a patient's life can become unbearably lonely and how they yearn for a normal life—a life in which someone does not notice the self-murmuring or the constant tendencies that set them apart from the rest of society. As a newly graduated nurse, I will continue to learn and educate myself about this illness and will strive to understand these patients in order to help educate others in forming better perceptions of schizophrenia.

Kathleen Nguyen, BSN, RN

Ms. Coughlan's and Ms. Nguyen's writings are reflective not only of the perceptions of new nurses and students, but also of more experienced nurses. They all speak of how their fear was based on the stigma of mental illness and influenced by what they have seen in movies, the news, and on television. I have always been aware of the societal stigma attached to schizophrenia, but working with student nurses and new graduates has opened my eyes to the fact that healthcare providers also place a stigma on these patients. Along with the responsibility of educating new nurses as well as managing a psychiatric unit comes the responsibility to decrease the stigma created by health care professionals about schizophrenia, a responsibility that I am eager to take on to ensure that those who suffer from schizophrenia receive the quality health care that they deserve.

Catherine Giasson, MSN, RN
Nurse Manager, Acute Psychiatry
VA Boston Health Care System

NOTE FROM THE AUTHOR

The inspiring story of Brandon Staglin's life to date is one that can be held up as a role model for those people who suffer from schizophrenia in that he, like others, with the support of his family, was able to recover from this serious illness and go on to help others so inflicted.

The story of Scott as written by his twin sister, Cyndi, one of my colleagues, exemplifies how the typical life begins for a person with schizophrenia. Until early adulthood, they have the interests, hopes, and aspirations of so many youth of their generation. Although Scott and Brandon had many advantages when they first became ill, too often other patients are lost to treatment in the current U.S. mental healthcare system that is governed by insurance policies and overworked caregivers. Adequate, intensive follow-up care is sometimes not given to those who clearly need it, particularly early in the illness course after first being diagnosed, partly because they do not recognize their need for it. Thus, patients can slip by with warning signs unnoticed. It is often left to families to take on this responsibility of knowing early enough when their relative is slipping into another episode of illness. Unfortunately, some patients are not lucky enough to have family members who stay supportive during the periods of evolving "strange" behavior such as that described by Brandon Staglin or Dr. Shannon-Weickert.

The perspective here of one nurse, Catherine, who has dedicated her life to helping people with mental illness, states clearly both the frustrations and rewards that come with her work, a service that is too often unnoticed by the public in general, families of patients, and the community of professionals. Many of the patients she sees are at the other end of the spectrum, those patients who are already chronic and have gone through multiple hospitalizations and treatment regimens and are often abandoned by their families and other support networks. They are considered "end stage" by too many mental care workers who by this time have given up hope for rehabilitating them. I call these patients "the forgotten" because too often the focus is on the beginning stages of illness, i.e., early detection and treatment both in the research and clinical worlds. However, the quality of life of those who have had persistent illness for many years should not be ignored. This is an illness that is not likely to be eradicated for years to come. Thus, we all continue to work toward achieving public recognition that schizophrenia is a medical disease and not some scary, unknown behavior to stigmatize, and that parity for mental illness in the healthcare system is necessary for improving the quality of care for these patients so that no one patient or family of a patient needlessly suffers. In addition, we continue to focus on developing new and better treatments, so that ultimately the "end stage" described in these "forgotten" ones that exists today on the chronic hospital psychiatric wards worldwide will be preventable.

Lynn Eleanor DeLisi, MD
Brockton, Massachusetts
February 12, 2016

INTRODUCTION

A patient recently slipped this poem as a message into my box. She said she wrote this for me and requested that it appear in this book with her name attached:

> *"I want to listen, but*
> *Do you hear?*
> *Was I taught by example*
> *Or by fear?*
> *How do I respond, when,*
> *I don't think I know?*
> *I lost it to circumstances,*
> *Out of my control.*
> *I was in the middle,*
> *Graphology would show.*
> *Made to be someone,*
> *I didn't even know.*
>
> Mary Lambert
> March 25,2015

I believe this poem says it all and illustrates the importance of compassionately caring for patients with schizophrenia and aiming to lead them to recovery.

I always knew that I would someday want to do something to inform the public about my experiences treating people with schizophrenia and investigating the causes and treatments of the illness in my own research. There seems to be a huge gap between the facts I know about this illness, and what the public perceives about schizophrenia. I still hear educated news broadcasters speak about inconsistent or split decisions in politics or world events as something that is "schizophrenic." This is reminiscent of a time in the 1980s, when my daughter came home from high school and told me her health teacher described schizophrenia as "split personality." I knew this statement was incorrect. Schizophrenia has long been thought of by the public as a "Jekyll and Hyde" type of condition, but this could not be farther from the truth. Yet for some reason psychiatrists have not been able to correct this misunderstanding.

When Bleuler coined the term "schizophrenia" in 1911, he erroneously used the Latin for "split mind." What he *meant* was that there was a "split"—or inconsistency—between the affect and emotions, thought and speech, and perhaps perception and reality. Unfortunately, what we name a condition can have repercussions for many years into the future. Someday, perhaps, the name of this illness (or set of illnesses) may change to something more reflective of the underlying biology, and it will be the biological changes that drive the classification of psychiatric disorders in general, not the clustering of clinical symptoms by themselves.

Nevertheless, the term schizophrenia has continued over the years to describe a psychiatric disorder that is very heterogeneous in its expression, clinical course, and biology. It has had an unusual course in social history. At the turn of the century, patients with these symptoms were shunned by society and isolated in large, gated multi-building complexes called psychiatric hospitals or institutions, often being committed there by relatives and staying for years — or for life. During World War II, the Nazi extermination policy began with a focus on patients in psychiatric hospitals, as they were deemed unfit to live and use a share of limited national resources. Many psychiatrists even played terrible roles in facilitating these policies because of their lack of understanding of the biology and inheritance of the disorder.

It was only in the late 1960s, when neuroleptic medications were accepted as the treatment of choice and marked improvement in behavior could be seen, that patients with schizophrenia were rehabilitated back into the community. Slowly, the public institutions were emptied, and residences sprang up within towns for patients who were stabilized and were treatable on an outpatient basis in the community. Periodically, questions about the nature of this illness resurface when someone with schizophrenia is in the news for having performed a violent act toward an innocent person or persons—then the prudence of releasing some patients prematurely from long-term hospital commitment is questioned.

One such famous case was John Hinkley, Jr., the young man who shot former president Reagan and one of his cabinet members (James Brady, who became permanently disabled as a result of this attack). He still is occasionally in the news as his illness has stabilized; he has aged, and is out in the community (supervised) for considerable lengths of time. Of course, many more violent crimes are committed by people who do *not* have the diagnosis of schizophrenia than by those with the diagnosis, but nevertheless, unpredictable behavior is a frightening hallmark of unstabilized or undertreated symptoms of schizophrenia, particularly of the paranoid type. These behaviors, plus the bizarre and inappropriate nature of some of the symptoms, lead to dire social consequences with implications not only for whether someone seeks appropriate treatment, but also for how someone with this diagnosis is viewed by people with whom he or she interacts socially, professionally, and legally. These characteristics led to the stigma that has been formed about schizophrenia over the years.

Unfortunately, because of the stigma attached to the disorder, physicians will often delay making a schizophrenia diagnosis and will then likely cause more damage by initially assuring parents that their son or daughter will "grow out of it." They may instead label the emotional difficulties as an "adjustment reaction," which requires no medication, but simply observation and psychotherapy over time. The harm in this is that we now know it is likely that early pharmacologic treatment may prevent the severe, chronic, debilitating form of the illness.

The stigmatization associated with schizophrenia extends into further aspects of life. Insurance companies do not treat schizophrenia as a medical illness that needs treatment in the same way as pneumonia, for instance, or other ailments that originate below the head. Employers would likely eliminate anyone who wrote on a job application that he or she had been diagnosed with schizophrenia. Families keep it secret when one of their relatives is afflicted with this disorder because the stigma may contribute to a potential mate's reluctance to marry into such a family. As with a history of depression, having had schizophrenia in one's past is too often used against those individuals who do recover, so that they are unlikely to ever hold a government office or to succeed in ways that they could have were it not for their diagnosis. Even other healthcare professional tend to be biased against providing comprehensive care to someone who is known to have schizophrenia and consider medical problems they are having either secondary to their psychiatric condition or the medications they take for it. We hope with education, this discrimination will eventually disappear.

Many famous and creative figures have been said to have had schizophrenia, or at least a psychotic illness that at times was certainly indistinguishable from schizophrenia. Among them are musicians (such as Brian Wilson from the Beach Boys), artists (Van Gogh), Nobel Prize winners (John Nash), kings (Christian VII of Denmark in the late 1700s), and revered historical figures such as Joan of Arc. They contrast at an extreme with other individuals diagnosed with this disorder, such as the Unabomber or the Yorkshire Ripper. Famous movies have depicted people with schizophrenia for decades, from the early horrors in *The Snake Pit*, to *One Flew Over the Cookoo's Nest*, to *I Never Promised You a Rose Garden*, *A Beautiful Mind* and *Changeling*. The latter film was particularly damaging, in that Angelina Jolie played a single mother whose child disappears. The police were less than sympathetic toward her and ultimately put her away in a mental institution, where she was treated for speaking out as if she had symptoms of paranoid schizophrenia and was met with a lack of compassion and nastiness from nurses, orderlies, and doctors. Any potential psychiatric patient who saw this 2008 movie would have likely not sought help for fear of being similarly mistreated.

Although some people aid in quelling the stigma surrounding this illness, others still point their fingers at people with schizophrenia, considering them peculiar and using the words "cuckoo," "nuts," "crazy," or "loco" to describe their thoughts and behavior. Most people who stigmatize people with schizophrenia know little about the scientific basis for this illness and whether their prejudices make practical sense. Even using the term "schizophrenic" rather than describing someone as "a person with schizophrenia," can be seen as insulting. This book is designed to refute the basis for the stigma surrounding schizophrenia and to provide the public with a glimpse of what it is like to have this disorder, what causes it, how it can be treated, and how one can live a productive life when he, she, or a family member has schizophrenia.

Today, clinicians and leaders in mental health talk of the clear possibility that recovery can happen in a large portion of people diagnosed with schizophrenia. The National Institutes of Mental Health (NIMH) invested a large amount of funds into working on a recovery plan for people first diagnosed with schizophrenia. This is called the RAISE project, something talked about further in this book. It was a huge success in establishing a standard for treatment that can lead to recovery and provides great hope for the future care of individuals with this diagnosis. Indeed, some very famous people with schizophrenia are said to have recovered, such as the author and attorney Elyn Saks, and the Nobel Prize winner, John Nash, both of whom were able to describe their recovery process in writing and speeches. At the time of the publication of this edition of *100 Questions & Answers About Schizophrenia*, John Nash had unfortunately passed away in an automotive accident. His example of successfully living with schizophrenia and recovering, however, will surely live on.

Lynn Eleanor DeLisi, MD
October 2015

PART 1

The Illness and Its Characteristics

"Mental pain is less dramatic than physical pain, but it is more common and also more hard to bear."

—CS Lewis (Healthyplace.com)

What is schizophrenia?

What are the first signs of this illness? How do I know whether someone has schizophrenia?

Is being "schizophreniform" the same as having "schizophrenia"?

More...

1. What is schizophrenia?

The word *schizophrenia* is clearly a misnomer. People with this disorder do not have a "split personality," as the word implies. Eugen Bleuler, who coined this term back in the early part of the 20th century, did so because he saw an abnormal "split" between the outward **affect** of the patient and his or her emotions, as well as a split between thought, speech, and affect. The split is actually due to an underlying misconnection of brain functional activity. A true split personality is quite a rare syndrome whereby a person assumes different identities; an environmental trigger initiates this switch. Usually these identities have been manifest in the mind of such an individual because of traumatic events, such as sexual abuse, having taken place in his or her childhood that have been extremely stressful to acknowledge. These individuals may benefit from intense psychotherapy over the years but are in no way similar clinically or biologically to people with schizophrenia.

Affect
The combination of body language, facial expression, and reactivity that signals an individual's engagement and awareness of the world around him or her.

Delusion
A false belief based on faulty judgment about one's environment.

Hallucination
Experiencing something from any of the five senses that actually is not occurring in reality.

DSM-5
The diagnostic and statistical manual developed by leading clinical psychiatrists in the United States for the systematic evaluation of psychiatric patients and assigning diagnoses to groups of symptoms. There have been five major separate revisions of this code of diagnoses since its inception.

Not only is the name misleading as above, but it leads to stigmatization of people with schizophrenia. Many well-meaning people use the abbreviated term "schizo" to describe anyone who behaves in a strange way or seems to be inconsistent or "split". Some people are starting movements in different parts of the world to change the name of this disorder to something with a more meaningful connotation. This change, however, remains in the future.

The American Psychiatric Association defines schizophrenia as a disorder consisting of **delusions** (see Question 10), **hallucinations**, disorganized speech, grossly disorganized/bizarre behavior, and/or a lack of organized speech, activity, or emotions (**DSM-5**, 2014) with active symptoms for at least one month. Usually at least two of these sets of symptoms are present. The illness begins with a prodromal stage, and after treatment or an acute episode subsides may be in a so-called "**residual**" stage, both having some often nonspecific behavioral symptoms. At least six months with continuous signs of some disturbance should be present. During this period, an individual with schizophrenia is clearly considered impaired in his or her ability to perform at work, attend school, or participate in social activities in a productive way. Criterion A lists the five key symptoms of psychotic disorders: (1) hallucinations, (2) delusions (see Question 10), (3) disorganized speech, (4) disorganized or catatonic behavior (see Question 9), and (5) negative symptoms (see Question 11). Two of these 5 symptoms are required, and at least one symptom must be delusions, hallucinations, or disorganized speech.

Residual

Having some nonspecific symptoms (usually negative symptoms), but no longer active psychotic ones.

The American Psychiatric Association (APA) has produced 5 different sets of diagnostic criteria for psychiatric disorders over the past 50 years (DSM-I through 5) and has been modifying the criteria for specific disorders for each new set published. Despite this, the debates between clinicians about what is or is not part of the schizophrenia diagnosis for each new DSM was not based on specific biological tests or diagnostic signs with illness specificity, but rather a clustering of clinical symptoms that together form an entity upon which a consensus of senior psychiatrists can agree. There recently has been an important movement under the leadership of the National Institutes of Mental Health (NIMH) in the United States to think of psychiatric illnesses as domains with uniform biological anomalies (the Research Domain Criteria or RDoC concept). The reasoning is that many of the clinical symptoms of mental illnesses overlap, and thus the underlying biology of the symptoms are more important for determining appropriate treatment than the categorical diagnosis itself. However, this new method of disease classification is not yet ready for clinical applications and is currently a concept on which future research studies can be based.

Auditory

Something that is experienced through hearing. Some schizophrenia patients have hallucinations consisting of voices speaking to them, known as auditory hallucinations.

Olfactory

Something that is experienced as an odor or scent. Some schizophrenia patients have described hallucinations that are odors.

One of the major symptoms of schizophrenia, the hallucinations, are most often **auditory**, although visual, **olfactory**, and tactile hallucinations have been described as well. The latter, however, are more often due to substance abuse (alcohol or street drugs) than schizophrenia when they predominate. The auditory hallucinations that distinguish schizophrenia are not just sounds: They are words spoken aloud as if someone else is actually speaking them, although no one is there. The "speaker" can be one person who is or is not recognized by the individual, and that person is commenting in some way on the hearer's behavior. Or there also can be multiple voices talking about the hearer, usually in a frightening or derogatory manner. Sometimes the hallucinations have been occurring for years before any other symptoms occur; they may be unrecognized by the individual as anything that is abnormal or not happening to everyone. Many times, when severe, they intrude into the person's life and daily activities. The patient can be found actually responding to the voices as if in conversation. Without experience, any examiner might have difficulty imagining what hallucinations are like.

The second type of symptom involves having delusions. The word *delusion* is certainly common, but the delusions of schizophrenia are sometimes characteristic. Many are bizarre to the normal person. For example, feeling that some unknown force is controlling one's actions or emotions or seeing objects in the environment with new meaning are delusions frequently mentioned by patients.

Similarly, one could be watching television or a movie and feeling that the people on the screen are giving the watcher some special messages. Common environmental situations, such as water dripping from a faucet, take on a new magical meaning. The feeling that parts of one's body are not one's own are described, as well as feeling like an actor on the "stage of life" and not being "real." Other common symptoms are the patient's belief that he or she has the ability to mind-read or the reverse feeling that other people know the patient's own thoughts, as if they are spoken on a loudspeaker. Patients with schizophrenia are often suspicious that people are harming them (e.g., by food poisoning) or that a complicated plot by the government against the individual is occurring.

These latter **paranoid** delusions may be accompanied by delusions of grandeur (thinking that one is or can have extraordinary powers or abilities that are in reality not possessed) and hyper-religiosity—that is, the idea that God has singled one out for a special mission. I once had a patient who knew he would "be president of the United States" because "God had told him." This was, however, someone who had been barely an average student throughout school and thought that London, England, was in the midwestern United States!

Paranoid

The delusional belief that people or organizations are attempting to harm one.

The third type of symptom, **disorganized speech**, is reflective of what is occurring within the "mind" of the individual and his/her thinking pattern. Thus, schizophrenia is often referred to by psychiatrists as "a formal thought disorder." Disorganized speech characteristically is speech that is hard to follow because the topic keeps shifting from one thing to another, and there appears to be no clear progression to the phrases or organization. The terms used to describe such speech is "**tangential**" when the speech wanders and never

Disorganized speech

Speech that is difficult to follow because topics and phrases change unexpectedly.

Tangential

Speech that wanders from subject to subject and does not return to the starting theme.

seems to come back to the original theme, while in "**circumstantial**" speech, eventually the original topic is completed. An example might be: "You asked me if I have relatives? I would like to write about my Aunt, who you know lives with John. My teacher, James, often scolds me. I don't listen to the math. There is a contest on TV you know that shows 2 boys and a girl. Mary is the girl who laughs...".

Circumstantial

Wandering speech that eventually returns to its original subject.

With regard to **grossly disorganized behavior**, one might observe that the individual is dressed strangely, i.e., wearing clothes inside out or layered haphazardly, or clothes that are shabby or inappropriate for the environment and weather. The individual may be living in disarray in his/her surroundings and clearly demonstrate a lack of self-care, with unkempt hair and unwashed body. His/her behavior may also seem bizarre: For example, a person with schizophrenia may be observed carrying inappropriate things on the street or walking down the center of a road rather than on a sidewalk, singing in a store and talking aloud to himself/herself. Some of these behaviors obviously can be risky, and such individuals often come to the attention of law enforcement agents, who then pick them up and bring them to a hospital. Others, however, simply become homeless and are not seen as bizarre in the context of other homeless individuals.

Grossly disorganized behavior

Behavior characterized by multiple factors, such as lack of self-care, unkempt clothing, strange or bizarre speech and other socially inappropriate aspects.

Most psychiatrists today would agree that schizophrenia is defined by at least three separate sets of symptoms: (1) positive ones that include hallucinations and delusions; (2) negative ones that include a general appearance of being flat (without much emotion), called "**flat affect**," withdrawal, a lack of much speech (or at least speech that is so general that it doesn't say anything), slowness

Flat affect

The appearance of being without emotion.

of movements and the appearance of slowness to thinking; and (3) a set of symptoms related to general disorganization (i.e., speech that is mixed-up or not getting to the point and behavioral disorganization). The latter is now considered a third cluster, defined as a disorganization syndrome.

Subtypes of schizophrenia and different types of related diagnoses exist as well. The paranoid subtype is marked by more frequent delusions and hallucinations rather than any disorganization, and the delusions are often paranoid in nature, but not always. The disorganized subtype most prominently displays the disorganization symptoms already mentioned. The catatonic subtype focuses on predominantly motor and speech changes that are either excessive or suboptimal. The undifferentiated subtype is generally a mixture of the others, with no one type being more prominent. Finally, the residual subtype is one in which the patient has become stabilized and no longer has the delusions and hallucinations but still does not seem normal and has many so-called negative symptoms (appearing withdrawn, speaking minimally, lacking initiative, etc.) that have not resolved. Note that these subtypes, however, are no longer used in the DSM-5. This is probably because they appear generally unreliable and subjective; that is different clinicians may assign patients to different subtypes, and over time, the subtypes may change in any given patient. Catatonia is no longer considered a subtype of schizophrenia, but rather it is a syndrome that can also appear in other psychiatric disturbances such as in the affective disorders.

2. What are the first signs of this illness? How do I know whether someone has schizophrenia?

The following cases illustrate the essence of this question:

Maryanne was a first-year medical student who received an educational loan that covered only the subsidized housing development in which she was forced to live. Prior to attending medical school, she grew up in a small midwestern town where her parents were shop owners who barely made ends meet. She was a shy child who read a lot and did very well in school; thus she was eventually accepted to medical school with a scholarship after completing a degree at a local college while living at home. When enrolled in medical school, she took a job as a waitress in a nearby bar during hours when she was not on call in the evening. She gained support from a group of female classmates and would often study with them in afternoons after class or during lunch breaks. Tension was high during exams, and classmate support was often emotionally helpful. Occasionally, marijuana was passed from student to student during mass cramming sessions and sometimes after smoking heavily, Maryanne would complain about other people and become anxious about some private problems she refused to discuss. Laurie, a fellow classmate, noticed at some point that Maryanne was occasionally, and then more frequently, missing classes. Finally, she and three other friends made the trip across town to Maryanne's apartment. The lights were dim, and at first their knocks went unheard. The students overheard chanting, however, and they persisted. Eventually, Maryanne came to the door dressed in bizarre, multicolored robes. Candles glowed in a circle surrounding her living room, and food and other items were scattered across the floor.

Maryanne explained that she had taken up meditating and was just practicing "mindfulness." She assured her friends that she was fine, but preferred to stay home that day. Eventually, when school administrators noticed her absence, she was called in and required to attend psychotherapy in order to return to school. Instead, she dropped out of school and disappeared.

Maryanne became unemployed and lost her apartment; she became homeless for a time, camping out in the woods in summer months. Finally, her parents were able to locate her and convince her to travel in their car to a psychiatric emergency room, where she was assessed, found to be in need of treatment, and hospitalized.

Robert was a 21-year-old high school graduate who played the guitar nights and weekends doing small gigs at local hang-outs and worked on construction jobs when he could get them during the day. He had a disadvantaged childhood, his parents having divorced when he was only 6. He lived with his father, but eventually moved out of his father's home when he was 18 to live with friends after his father took on a new live-in girlfriend. He and his friends spent many hours smoking marijuana when not working, and Robert, who had many anxieties about being able to mix well in social situations, began to use marijuana more frequently, until his use became daily at least 3 times per day. He then began fighting with his roommates and began thinking they were stealing his things, to the point where he became convinced that they broke his computer codes and were spying on him through Facebook and Twitter and special cameras hidden in his computer and iPhone. He eventually moved out, but because of his need to continue using marijuana daily, he was also working less and less. The weather was warm at this time, so he began sleeping on park benches. Sometimes he would lie awake on a bench, staring at the stars; he started hearing voices that emanated from them as if people in "Heaven" were talking to him and telling him what to do. He received a text message from a friend he hadn't seen in several months asking where he was, but he thought the message actually came from God, who was trying to communicate with him. One day, he stole some new clothing from a local Walmart and began changing his clothes by the park bench. A passer-by became alarmed and called the police, who arrested him and placed him in jail overnight. By the time he appeared before a judge with his court appointed attorney, he appeared disheveled and was talking to himself. When the judge asked him if he understood what he was being charged with, his response was unrelated to the question and focused on the codes on his computer having been violated. Luckily, this judge was sensitive to the signs of mental illness and transferred him to a local public psychiatric facility for a full evaluation. Once seen by psychiatrists, he responded well to educational sessions, participated in substance abuse therapy groups, and worked with a team comprised of a psychiatrist, a psychologist, and a social worker, all of whom provided him with treatment and placement into available programs in the community. Even supportive work therapy was available to him so that he could get back to earning his own funds. His prognosis was fairly good, provided he recognized that he had developed a schizophrenia-like illness, that he needed to terminate his marijuana use, and that he would need to regularly and consistently take medication for some time (see **Part 2** for discussion of how long).

Another illustration is the case of Kevin, who grew up in a family with a long military legacy. His paternal great-grandfather fought in World War II, and family legend said that he was a hero rescuing fellow comrades on the Normandy beaches on D-Day. Despite this, when he returned home, he eventually had difficulties adjusting to civilian life and for a long time heard voices of dying soldiers and was worried about the enemy coming after him. One time he was hospitalized in a state facility for about 6 months, but no one in the family knew the details. Eventually, he recovered, married, and had a family that included Kevin's father. Kevin's father was an officer in the marines and fought in Vietnam. It was therefore always presumed that Kevin would join the armed services. Growing up in a very strict household with 2 older sisters, he could never measure up to their academic achievements and was periodically punished by beatings with a belt whenever he came home from school with grades that his parents thought were below his capacity. His teachers were concerned about his lack of attention in school, disorganized presentation, and inability to sit still for long and listen to the day's lessons. He eventually was tested by a psychologist at age 8 and thought to have **attention deficit hyperactivity disorder (ADHD)**, which was treated with Ritalin until Kevin was 15. During his teen years, he seemed to be bullied frequently by his fellow classmates because he had gained weight and was awkward in sports. At times, he would enter his home crying and be comforted by his older sisters. He rarely invited others over his home to "hang out" and only had one friend, a girl who was also bullied by others. He would usually sit for long hours in his room playing a guitar, which he had become quite adept at, but he avoided playing for other people and avoided mixing with friends. Kevin developed fears of going to large, crowded department stores or malls, and when he was in such places, he would have the feeling that people were laughing at him and noticing his strange appearance. He was never interested in having an iPhone or being

Attention deficit hyperactivity disorder (ADHD)

A neurological disorder characterized by inattentiveness and inability to focus.

able to text other people for communication and feared that if he carried a phone, too many people would be able to track him. He did have a computer, though, and would isolate himself for hours at a time playing games that would generally kill off fictitious characters on the screen. His parents assumed that he would just "grow out of" these behaviors and thought the Army might be good for him and would help him mature, so after graduation, he enlisted in the Army and was sent off to basic training. The rigors of basic training combined with the close interpersonal environment caused much stress for Kevin. Towards the end of his 6 weeks of training, he was found curled up in a guard tower in his underwear and unable to speak. An emergency medical team was called to retrieve him and he was then hospitalized at a military hospital, where he was diagnosed with "catatonia" (see Question 9).

Stories such as Maryanne's, Robert's, and Kevin's are all too common, although the outcome can go several different ways, largely depending on the supports individuals have within the community and whether their symptoms are detected early enough to be brought to the attention of mental healthcare professionals who can divert them into the appropriate treatment programs. These three individuals had in common a long period of nonspecific symptoms that in retrospect might be considered the **prodrome** to schizophrenia. A history of ADD or ADHD is frequently found in the childhood histories of individuals who eventually develop schizophrenia, as are childhood traumas of various types and a family history of some form of serious mental illness.

Prodrome

An early or premonitory symptom of a disease. If true specific prodromal symptoms are known, one can detect the illness early. These symptoms signify that the disease will be almost certain.

Since schizophrenia begins frequently when someone is in early adulthood, it can lead to a cessation of normal life and a loss of the potential the patient's future held as a young adult. Often relatives and close friends are unaware of why the individual is wary of confiding in anyone and remains reclusive or hard to find. The person who is developing schizophrenia rarely has any insight that he or she is ill and thus does not admit to anyone that they have stressful thoughts and perceptions occurring, despite their disturbing nature, nor do they seek help. Those who are close—friends and relatives—may notice a change in behavior and emotional responses; however, they do not know that the affected person is having hallucinations and delusionary thoughts unless the person says things that sound bizarre or that clearly cannot be true. More often, particularly when delusions are of a paranoid nature, these things are kept to oneself. Family and friends often think the problem can be fixed by encouraging the individual to "change scenery" by joining the military or traveling abroad. Families, if intact, frequently will rally to support the ill individual after recognizing problems, but often do not think that the person needs professional help unless the behavior becomes extreme. Once they do obtain help for their sick relative, as time goes by, they may eventually be depleted of funds and frustrated by the lack of community and legal support to aid their relative. Parents may eventually become resigned to caring for their child with schizophrenia permanently, but as they age, they worry about who will care for the child after they are gone. Support groups for families of people with mental illness have been very helpful for advice, and these will be discussed elsewhere. The focus recently in most of the industrialized nations has been on early detection of the signs that precede schizophrenia (the prodrome) and educating teachers, primary care doctors, and the public about when they should seek further professional help. It is hoped that by doing this, the long-term outcome for these individuals will be complete recovery and some of the misconceptions mentioned below will not happen.

Psychiatric researchers continuously debate about how best to predict that a schizophrenia-like illness is likely to occur. It would be important to find clear predictors that can distinguish the symptoms of illness from the variation in functioning and the "ups and downs" of stages of life experiences, particularly in adolescence. No clear predictors, however, have been found. The key probably has to do with change from one's usual functioning (i.e., withdrawal from friendships, peculiar statements that are not true, and a change in organization of behavior and speech). Work and school activities change for the worse, and an overall troubled withdrawal of the individual becomes apparent to those with whom he or she interacts. This individual may be heard talking to himself or herself or making untrue or bizarre statements about other people or events. Marijuana and other drug use can accelerate this process. The signs and symptoms often reach the point at which the individual behaves in an inappropriate or harmful manner (such as undressing in public or walking down the middle of a highway). In other instances, the individual will perform impulsive and aggressive acts without understanding the consequence of such actions. At this point the police are called, and the individual is brought to either jail or a psychiatric emergency room. Obviously, it is beneficial if early signs can be recognized and treated before they develop into a dangerous situation.

Depression

A major psychiatric condition characterized by profound sadness all day. It is usually accompanied by physical symptoms, such as loss of appetite, loss of sleep, and slowness in movements and speech.

Generally, schizophrenia develops gradually, on average over about a two-year period in an adolescent or young adult with behavioral changes from whatever his or her baseline was—such as withdrawing more than usual socially, a noticeable decline in academic performance, a new irritability, or what appears as **depression** (see Question 13)—and these are first noticed by close friends or family. Such individuals may also be found sleeping either too much or too little and are periodically agitated. These things might eventually lead a parent to consult a family physician about his or her child. The parent might be told that "adolescent turmoil" or "adjustment problems" are the cause. Most physicians have been delaying making a diagnosis of schizophrenia, particularly if the patient does not admit to clear auditory hallucinations and bizarre delusions. The **stigma** of having this disorder is still great (see Question 97), and the misperceived notion that it is like a "cancer of the mind" that lasts a lifetime is a "death sentence" that no physician wants to give unless he/she can no longer avoid it. The message to a parent may simply be that their son or daughter will "grow out of it," but at least with frequent follow-up appointments the patient may eventually admit to clear symptoms, which gives the opportunity for early treatment and possible prevention of the severe, chronic form of the illness. The typical new case, however, continues to be a young person who has done something clearly bizarre and harmful either to himself/herself or to others, which is generally the point where the police or a psychiatric crisis unit is called for help. In at least half of the cases in several countries, some kind of street drug use may be acutely responsible for (or at least contribute to) the bizarre and harmful behavior when it becomes a crisis. Many first-episode patients, after being treated and having the symptoms resolve, conclude that drug use was the cause and that they will be okay as long as they abstain from drugs (see **Part 5** for a more detailed discussion of drug abuse). This assumption, however, is false in many cases. The drugs may have initiated the disease that might have eventually occurred regardless. The danger is that the patient will assume that as long as street drugs are not taken again, he or she does not need the **neuroleptic** medication prescribed. Often, patients who make this assumption terminate the medications and treatment

Stigma

Literally a "mark"; something visible to others that sets an individual apart from others whether for justified or unjustified reasons.

Neuroleptic

Any medication that when given to animals will cause catalepsy. This name then was used to label all drugs that had an effect on reducing the symptoms of schizophrenia. In the past, neuroleptics were known as the "major tranquilizers", but the latter term is rarely used.

given during the acute episode, and the patient eventually **relapses** and comes back to the hospital in a more serious condition, with symptoms that are generally more difficult to suppress with medication. Patients who terminate their first treatment without being integrated into the chronic care system are most likely to be at high risk for suicide, and thus great efforts should be made to engage such patients and their families in programs for support and treatment.

Relapse

A recurrence of overt illness in a patient who previously had been stabilized.

As can be seen, stigma—both by the general public and physicians who diagnose and do the treating—is a serious problem that will need to be conquered if this disorder is to be identified early and treated aggressively before chronic deterioration sets in.

3. Is being "schizophreniform" the same as having "schizophrenia"?

In **schizophreniform disorder**, a patient has all the symptoms of schizophrenia, but the symptoms resolve in less than 6 months without residual effects remaining. Generally, this person was functioning very well and very suddenly developed symptoms that also resolved relatively quickly, with or without medication. However, someone may initially be diagnosed as "schizophreniform," but after 6 months' time the illness evolves into a clear diagnosis of schizophrenia; that is, even if medications are effective in suppressing most symptoms, some symptoms remain, and the doctor feels it is in the best interest of the patient to continue on medication. The majority of people who have a diagnosis of schizophreniform disorder eventually are diagnosed as having schizophrenia.

Schizophreniform disorder

Having the symptoms of schizophrenia, but over too short a period of time (less than 6 months) to be called schizophrenia.

4. What does it mean to have a "schizotypal personality disorder"?

There are mild forms of schizophrenia that sometimes are present in family members of people who have schizophrenia. Sometimes they are just referred to as the "spectrum" disorders and other times as "**schizotypal personality disorder**." This refers to specific traits that make one stand out and are often thought of as peculiar by other people observing them. Speech that is "stilted"—too formal for the specific conversation—or unfocused and rambling is characteristic of schizotypal personality disorder. Someone who is characterized as schizotypal may believe in things like extrasensory perception (ESP), horoscope predictions, or superstitions; have strange feelings and misperceptions of things they see and hear from time to time; feel paranoid and suspicious of others beyond reason; have few friends and refuse to socialize; or live alone in peculiar or bizarre circumstances. These are traits that might be stable over time and characteristic of the person. They sometimes, but not always, interfere with leading a "normal" life depending on the occupation and living circumstances of the individual. For example, everyone has at one time or another noticed an acquaintance or someone in the neighborhood who appears peculiar, dresses strangely, and hoards stacks of newspapers piled high in his/her house, as well as collections of other objects; or one might see or hear about another neighbor with 9 cats and known to live in the dark with curtains drawn during the day.

Schizotypal personality disorder

Specific traits that are considered unusual, e.g., odd speech patterns, in a person who may not have schizophrenia.

Many of the traits of schizotypal personality disorder can also be interchanged with paranoid and schizoid personality disorders, the former mainly a disorder of unreasonable or distorted suspicion about others, and

Schizoaffective disorder

Having both prominent symptoms of schizophrenia and depression and/or mania that overlap with the schizophrenia-like symptoms. However they do not always coincide so that sometimes the patients has only schizophrenia-like symptoms and other times, although less so, only mania or depressive symptoms.

Psychosis

Loss of connection with reality; experiencing delusions (i.e., false beliefs), and hallucinations. Psychotic persons often exhibit bizarre and risky behavior and do not seem to be aware that they are doing anything unusual.

Mania

A state of heightened arousal characterized by excessive emotion, e.g., elation, anxiety, fear, anger, or irritability. Behavior is characterized by fast speech and thoughts, agitation, reduced need for speech, feeling "on top of the world", and sometimes performing bizarre or risky actions.

the latter a disorder of social withdrawal and a preference to be by one's self. Each emphasizes different types of traits, but are frequently related, and all can present in the same individual. While these may never progress to clear schizophrenia, in some instances having these charachteristics may also be considered part of the prodrome to schizophrenia.

Treatment (if sought) for schizotypal disorder varies; it depends on whether the individual seeks help to change his/her life in some way and is also symptom-specific. Sometimes a low dose of risperidone or other second-generation antipsychotic medication is known to alleviate symptoms relating to language and thought disorganization, as well as suspiciousness and misperceptions. Sometimes the symptoms of withdrawal may respond to an antidepressive medication, while the excessive social anxiety often present may respond to antianxiety medications. Psychotherapy and psychological therapies may also be helpful, either by itself or in combination with medication, specifically if it is focused on teaching the patient how to improve specific social skills and some behaviors that may offend or have negative impacts on others.

5. What is schizoaffective disorder?

Schizoaffective disorder is a diagnosis that forms a link between **psychosis** and mood and should only be made when it is difficult to distinguish whether a patient has schizophrenia or a mood disorder. *DSM-5* requires the mood episode (whether it is **mania**, depression, or both) to be present for the majority of the illness.However, it also requires that there be at least a 2-week period when the active symptoms of schizophrenia are present without a major depressive or manic episode present concurrently.

A patient with this disorder has all the symptoms of schizophrenia, but also has symptoms of depression, manic behavior, or both. Depression is generally defined as feeling very sad emotionally for at least a week at a time, withdrawing from friends and usual activities, feeling overwhelming guilt, perhaps to the point of having suicidal ideas or actions, with loss of weight, appetite, and sleep as a result. Manic behavior, on the other hand, is feeling excessively elated and cheery, with very fast speech and thoughts, not needing to sleep, and perhaps also doing some bizarre and risky acts during this period as well. Agitated behavior is sometimes seen with manic behavior. Grandiose delusions are also part of this syndrome.

Interestingly, psychiatrists generally differ in whether they would diagnose someone with schizophrenia or schizoaffective disorder, as well as any of the subtypes of schizophrenia, and over the course of illness in one individual these diagnoses seem to change, which is why it is not clear that they are really separate disorders. Similarly, psychiatrists sometimes differ in whether someone with schizoaffective disorder should at some times be diagnosed with **bipolar affective disorder** (also called manic-depression). The fact is that many of the symptoms overlap. Thus, patients are sometimes diagnosed with schizoaffective disorder yet may be diagnosed by different psychiatrists as having schizophrenia, while still others may regard them as having bipolar disorder.

Bipolar affective disorder

A psychiatric condition characterized by mood swings that occur episodically. Sometimes, particularly when very "high" (manic), people with bipolar disorder can have many of the characteristic positive symptoms of schizophrenia.

To date, it still remains unclear how valid this diagnostic category really is, and it is likely that many psychiatrists still use this diagnosis too often to classify their patients. Schizoaffective disorder may ultimately be found to be the same disorder as schizophrenia in its biologic origins.

Another view is that a biologic continuum likely exists between all these diagnoses. The extremes and more classical cases of each are more consistently diagnosable among different psychiatrists, but the vast majority fall into a spectrum of disorders, with the schizoaffective category being the middle. Patients who do not show "classic" symptoms of schizophrenia can either be called **schizophrenia-spectrum disorder**, or alternatively will be classified and treated according to the symptoms that occur, rather than the category of diagnosis. It may be that the underlying biology of what appear to be different illnesses may really be the same disease that is clinically expressed in varying ways in different individuals, from a very disorganized schizophrenia-like degenerative illness to a cyclic episode of psychotic symptoms with normality in between, the so-called "**unitary psychosis**" (Crow, 1990). Alternatively, there may be several biological causes, but their clinical manifestations may cross over the tradition clinical diagnostic boundaries that psychiatry has established. When we can clearly designate definitively related biological underpinnings (such as **genes** or their expression; see **Part 3**) for aspects of schizophrenia, it is anticipated that entirely different diagnostic categories may be developed that will then reflect the biology more directly.

Schizophrenia-spectrum disorder

An alternative name for patients with schizoaffective disorder who do not show the classic symptoms.

Unitary psychosis

The hypothesis that all schizophreniform disorders are biologically the same disease expressed differently in different individuals.

Gene

A functional unit of heredity that is in a fixed place in the structure of a chromosome.

In summary, currently, many people with a psychotic illness have been diagnosed with schizoaffective disorder because they may have psychosis (i.e., delusions and hallucinations), and when they present with an illness exacerbation, they frequently may have suicidal thoughts and feel "depressed" or be agitated with explosive anger that is difficult to separate from mania. At these times, they may be given an antidepressant, as well as a mood stabilizer. It is then often difficult for the next physician seeing this patient months later to decide whether the patient still needs these medications or a trial of discontinuing some of them is warranted (see **Part 2: Treatment**). It is the opinion of this writer that far too many patients receive the diagnosis of schizoaffective disorder and receive too many medications in combination; at some point each patient needs a new evaluation of his/her lifetime of illness course and symptoms as well as in medications, so in order that an appropriate treatment plan can be reinstituted.

6. How is schizophrenia different from manic depression or bipolar disease?

Although, as mentioned above, some research psychiatrists believe that a biological continuum exists between the extremes of these two disorders, there are differences. Many people with bipolar disorder can lead a normal, productive, and very creative life after their mood is stabilized and particularly if they have some insight that they have an illness and thus are compliant with their medication regime prescribed by a physician. In fact, before the full-blown illness, this person may be a high achiever and model citizen in his/her community and thus once the symptoms develop into a crisis, those around him/her are surprised and bewildered that they somehow missed that something was wrong. Consider Philip Haynes Markoff, the "Boston Craigslist Killer," notorious in the national news in the United States a few years ago. This was a medical student, a star by all criteria, who was socially very well-liked and academically performing very well. The only indication of anything wrong was that one person described him as "having mood swings." However, given the normal life stresses in this young man's life, mood changes would not be unusual. What was unusual was his bizarre and risky behavior that suddenly ensued: meeting massage therapists in hotels, hoarding their underwear, and finally shooting one with a gun that he had kept in a hollowed-out Gray's Anatomy textbook. This was not a usual criminal, but rather someone who clearly developed the onset of a psychotic disorder, likely bipolar, that unfortunately was not treated before his behavior became harmful to others. This story, although an extreme that made news headlines, is all too frequent. Nevertheless, after stabilization on medication and after such a manic episode, providing that medication is continued, individuals with this condition appear to retain their original potential for functioning. Cognitive abilities are not impaired, as they more often are in schizophrenia, and the individual may be able to go back to his/her normal life if he has not committed a crime during the acute stage of illness such as the medical student mentioned above.

There are many examples of very successful individuals with bipolar disorder who have been role models and inspirations for others with the illness, such as Dr. Kay Jamison, a professor at Johns Hopkins. Similarly, there are also many cases of schizophrenia, such as Elyn Saks, a professor, a dean and an attorney, who wrote about her illness in the book, *A Centre Cannot Hold;* and Brendan Staglin, who begins this book with his personal story, and who has become a successful communicator and supportive of efforts to combat mental illness. Many more examples could be cited.

There are also, however, more severe cases of bipolar disorder with several frequent hospitalizations that eventually are indistinguishable from chronic, severe schizophrenia.

In general, both the premorbid state (the time prior to illness onset) and the outcomes are what differ between schizophrenia and bipolar disorder, despite some of the biology and clinical symptoms being similar. Schizophrenia is more often thought of as a **neurodevelopmental** disorder with a poorer premorbid adjustment socially and academically in childhood, whereas pre-bipolar individuals are indistinguishable from others in those earlier years. For example, drawing again from national news stories, the Aurora, Colorado movie theatre and the Newtown, Connecticut elementary school shootings were completed by young men who were very disturbed and had untreated and slowly evolving cases of likely schizophrenia.

Neurodevelopmental

Happening during the growth and formation of different structures of the brain.

Much biologic research comparing the biology of these two disorders needs to be performed. Many of the brain structural changes present in schizophrenia have been found in bipolar disorder, although it is mainly severe bipolar disorder with psychotic features (such as hallucinations and delusions) that appears to show these changes.

7. Is it possible to hear voices that are not there and not be ill?

Recently, reports of surveys of the general population of people (those not seeking treatment) conclude that auditory hallucinations and various forms of delusions are more common than previously thought. In fact, the investigators of these studies report that psychotic experiences are present in anywhere from 5 to 20% of the general population. This statement needs to be interpreted with caution, however, because sufficient follow-up has not been done of the people reporting these experiences to know whether eventually they will be diagnosed with full-blown schizophrenia or another serious psychiatric disturbance.

Many psychiatrists who treat patients with schizophrenia find that their patients frequently admit to having heard voices as far back as they can remember in childhood and never thought to mention these experiences, as they weren't perceived to be "abnormal."

Having auditory hallucinations alone certainly does not mean that you have or will get schizophrenia. Many people never have any medical or psychiatric problems relating to the voices they hear, but instead have these experiences in relation to falling to sleep or just waking (not being fully alert) or may have them during illness with high fevers.

Another difference has to do with the nature of the voices. Hearing someone calling your name or hearing sounds but not complex language is less serious. The hallmarks of classical schizophrenia are hearing more than one voice having a conversation about the hearer and/or at least one voice commenting on the hearer's actions. There are also "**command hallucinations**," which give the hearer orders to carry out some action. These latter experiences are certainly more disturbing and characteristic of illness. They rarely stand alone, however, and are most often accompanied by either some form of bizarre behavior or multiple delusions.

Command hallucinations

Imaginary voices that tell the hearer what to do.

8. Does being told one has a psychosis mean one has schizophrenia?

Psychosis is a broader term than schizophrenia and implies that one is not in touch with reality, either because perceptual problems, such as auditory or visual hallucinations, are present or because they have beliefs that are not based on reality. When someone is thought to be "psychotic," they may not have all the designated criteria for schizophrenia. Some psychotic behavior is present at the height of mania, and can also be present at the very low point of a clear depression. In addition, psychosis may have other origins, such as substance abuse, hormonal disorders, vitamin deficiencies, or other chemical disorders, sometimes referred to as metabolic disturbances. Hyperthyroidism is often accompanied by psychosis, while hypothyroidism may more often be accompanied by depression; some neurodegenerative disorders, such as Parkinson's disease, **Alzheimer's disease** and Huntington's chorea, may have psychotic components, sometimes occurring long before the disorder itself is diagnosed. The autoimmune disorder, lupus erythematosus, can be mistakenly diagnosed as schizophrenia or an unknown psychosis. There are many other, relatively infrequent disorders that also have such similar presentations. Moreover, certain medications for the above and other conditions may also have psychotic symptoms as side effects. A good psychiatrist will carefully consider all these other potential diagnoses, particularly when they require specific treatments, when seeing someone with a psychosis for the first time.

Alzheimer's disease

This is one of a few progressive brain diseases that has been diagnosed in older people who appear disoriented and having difficulty communicating properly to others. A person with Alzheimer's disease has trouble remembering what happened 1 minute ago and has difficulty forming sentences and speaking, eventually progressing into not being able to take care of one's basic needs.

Catatonia

A condition that is characterized by extremes in behavior, of which the individual appears to be unaware. These behaviors include being mute or in a stupor and immobile to at the other extreme, being in an excitatory state of an extreme frenzy or agitated excitement.

9. What is catatonia?

Catatonic behavior is the extreme of disorganized behavior, and can involve either complete immobility and muteness or, at the opposite end, extreme, disorganized excitability—an extreme frenzy-like behavior. **Catatonia** in its full-blown syndrome is actually rare today in the United States and Western nations, although it can be seen more frequently in impoverished countries where patients do not get ample care and lack access to the newest pharmaceutical treatments available.

Patients with catatonia are often quite remarkable in their appearance. They have what has been termed "waxy flexibility"; that is, they stand in one position with their limbs stationary until a person moves them to another position, where they will stay until again moved by another person. Sometimes they are brought to emergency rooms and thought to be in a coma. However, they may quickly come out of it when given large doses of **benzodiazepines**, such as clonazepam, when catatonia is suspected. Although catatonia was generally thought to be a subtype of schizophrenia in the past, more careful approaches to understanding its presentation have led to the belief that it occurs in a variety of diagnoses, such as affective disorders, as well as schizophrenia, and is now considered a symptom state and not a diagnostic category. A currently practicing U.S. psychiatrist may never have seen such cases of catatonia because of their rarity.

Benzodiazepines
A class of medications used in the treatment of various psychiatric disorders.

Nevertheless, one patient I remember clearly from the mid 1980s (when catatonia was not often seen) was a young man who had driven himself to the outpatient clinic. After approaching the check-in desk, however, the receptionist looked up to find him immobile, stiff, and mute. I led him to a private room. He responded several minutes later, but only after having been administered a **tranquilizer** intramuscularly. He denied that anything unusual was happening and was aware that we were discussing him, but he had no explanation for why he had not responded. He then drove home without incident, but frequently entered my office again in that same manner.

Tranquilizer
Any drug that is used to calm or pacify an anxious and/or agitated person. Major tranquilizers are the class of drugs used for psychotic symptoms. These terms are not often used anymore.

I also recall a memorable experience when visiting the National Psychiatric Hospital in El Salvador in early 2001. Touring this hospital that was so ill-equipped compared with U.S. public psychiatric hospitals was a startling awakening to the reality of the status of current psychiatric care in impoverished developing countries. High doses of old medicines were used, as psychiatrists did not know that newer drugs existed. The floors of the wards had drains to collect the urine that often was uncontrollably produced. What mainly stood out, however, were the several immobile individuals with classical catatonic schizophrenia exhibiting pronounced waxy flexibility. More recently, as a hospital-based psychiatrist, another young man was admitted to my service from a medical unit where he was immobile and on intravenous-fluids. No medical work-up revealed any cause for this condition and he was breathing and his heart was found to be normal, as well as all his other organ systems. He was not in a coma, as his eyes were open and occasionally he looked around, although he failed to talk. EEG and MRI scans were normal. Neurologist ruled out that he had a stroke. We began giving him moderate doses of a benzodiazepine, and after 3 days he began slowly to talk to me, getting out of bed to go to meals. He denied anything was wrong with him, spoke in perfect speech without any delusions or abnormalities and insisted that he be discharged. I believe this was a catatonic episode and though I never saw this patient again, I assume that if untreated, he likely had other episodes afterwards with similar hospital stays. Unfortunately, we do not understand the biological mechanism that underlies this condition, and because it has become so rare over recent years, it is understudied.

10. What is a delusion?

A delusion is defined as a fixed, false belief that remains despite evidence to the contrary. Many times it is difficult to distinguish "real" delusions from cultural norms or outside stresses that are happening to individuals. For example, I once had a patient who worked as a secretary for the CIA. She claimed that her phone was "bugged" and people were following her. Was this a delusion, or could it have actually been happening because of the nature of her job? Having a third-party informant to clarify such situations may frequently be necessary.

Besides paranoid delusions, there are many classical ones that patients with schizophrenia often talk about: feeling that the commentators on the TV are talking directly to them; feeling that they are on a stage and everyone is acting as if this is not real life; thinking that people can hear their thoughts or that their thoughts are on a loudspeaker, as if broadcast; feeling that their thoughts are not their own and someone else has inserted them into their minds, or even that someone has taken their own thoughts out; that an external force is controlling his/her movements and actions. Other frequent delusions are feeling that one's dental fillings have transmitters attached that control one's mind or that someone has implanted metal into one's body that transmits radio waves. Sometimes the delusions are considered grandiose, such as believing that one is a movie star, or has a special mission that God has requested. Delusions can also be even more bizarre: For example, having a theory that is completely fictional about the origins and working of the universe or of how the brain works.

With respect to religious beliefs, sometimes it is particularly difficult to separate excessive religiosity from delusionary experiences. For example, several years ago, I worked not far from a revival church in which congregations would assemble and sing progressively louder, to a point where members were drawn into chanting trances, almost as if they had no control over their actions and were so overcome by the event that one could perceive that they were all in acute psychotic states. When the music stopped and the meeting was over, however, each individual returned to normal. Less extreme examples may be cultural beliefs about the powers of shamans, the healing powers of some preachers or "holy sites," etc. When religion interferes with one's social life, occupational and educational achievements, you can call the beliefs a "symptom" of a disorder. Certainly, this is one illustration that psychopathology is likely to be on a continuum in many ways between what is considered normal by society and what is considered abnormal by psychiatrists.

In past years, debates existed about whether schizophrenia actually exists other than in the imagination of psychiatrists. Although this view is certainly extreme, the cultural environment of a newly presenting patient needs to be considered before a diagnosis is made. The disorder that is described in this book is more than extreme views that can be related to culture. It affects individuals from all cultural backgrounds and races equally, and many of the delusions are more similar than they are different across cultures. How to separate "beliefs" that have no scientific proof from "delusions" that can be defined as pathological is a matter of philosophical debate that will undoubtedly continue over time. It is, however, beyond the scope of this book.

11. What is meant by positive and negative symptoms?

Positive symptoms

Considered the active symptoms of hallucinations and delusions of schizophrenia.

Negative symptoms

Those characteristics of psychiatric illness that present as withdrawn behavior, an expressionless face, a lack of initiative, a lack of interest, not saying much when talking and saying things in short sentences, lessened thoughts, and slowed movements.

Positive symptoms are those that produce activity. These are things that are said, acted on, or that clearly disturb the individual, such as delusions and hallucinations. **Negative symptoms** (the so-called defect state) are things that are lacking in activity or reduce it—thus, "negative." These include a lack of movement, speech, emotional expression, social ability, or initiative to do anything. Positive symptoms tend to fluctuate and respond better to current medications than negative symptoms. Negative symptoms are more stable over time and may be present in the beginning of the illness but are more manifest when the illness becomes chronic and can be the only signs of illness in the stabilized "residual" cases. It is thought that the newer "atypical" medications—particularly clozapine but also olanzapine, quetiapine, risperidone, and others—may have an effect on reducing negative symptoms, but carefully done research studies to date have failed to support this hypothesis. Sometimes, depressive symptoms can overlap with negative ones, and these are what may be improving. Since patients with schizophrenia can benefit from antidepressant medication for episodes of depression, these symptoms must also be carefully distinguished. Suicidal behavior has been found in some studies to be particularly reduced by clozapine treatment.

12. Do people with schizophrenia have language problems?

Frequently, a patient with schizophrenia who is in an acute state may speak in a very disorganized and loose manner, wherein sentences do not appear to be connected by logical meaning. For example, a typical utterance might be: "I just saw a man walk down the street to open the door. But why is he throwing the ball? Do you know where the soda bottle came from? Doctor, can you get me out of this jail?... " and so on. This kind of speech may be described as "circumstantial," "tangential," and/or having "flight of ideas," and is known as "the formal thought disorder" of schizophrenia. However, often patients with schizophrenia do not always speak in such obviously mixed-up fashion, but have more subtle peculiarities of language that can only be detected by specific types of psychological testing.

Nevertheless, regardless of whether the above is present, the major symptoms of schizophrenia can all be explained by an underlying disorder in the brain pathways that process language, both that which is perceived and that which is spoken. For example, the brain of someone with schizophrenia may have misconnections between the auditory centers and those parts of the brain that perceive language, so that the patient will misperceive what the speaker has actually said. This may be the origin of delusions.

Similarly, with misconnections between the language and speech centers of the brain, the resulting spoken words may seem garbled and possibly represent thought that is also disorganized because of misconnections in the brain. When the brain auditory pathways are misconnected in language centers, then it will appear that the patient is "hearing" his or her own thoughts or someone else speaking, when in fact no sounds are present. Thus, the disorganization of brain language pathways can more directly be seen as a symptom of these misconnections and can occur in the more severe cases. The negative symptoms of schizophrenia may be directly caused by language pathway deficits, such as in a lack of complex speech, a lack of content of speech, or a secondary result of the positive symptoms that are disturbing and preoccupying internally. The use of new brain imaging technology is helping researchers to make progress in delineating these connections in the brain, and while it remains unclear which specific brain connections are disturbed, great strides are now being made to map not only those for language, but those for being able to perceive emotion and facial expressions, as well as fear. In addition, new studies are focusing on the so-called "resting state" and what goes on in the mind of someone who has schizophrenia without any stimulation that is different from others.

Studies of children who later developed schizophrenia are interesting because some have been shown to have had a delay in the development of language, such that his or her first words occur later in time than most children and they are put into sentences even later. Learning to read is also delayed in these children to a varying degree. This slowing of the acquisition of the building blocks for language suggests abnormalities in the timing and construction of brain pathways for language.

13. Do people with schizophrenia get depression?

Depression is more commonly a characteristic symptom of schizophrenia than most clinicians have realized. In fact, the majority of patients with chronic schizophrenia have had an episode of being depressed at some time in the course of their illness. Often, the first onset of schizophrenia will be preceded by several months of what patients will describe as a depression. In addition, as an episode of acute schizophrenia resolves, depression may follow. Sometimes, however, depressive symptoms can be confused with negative symptoms of slower and less frequent speech, slowed movements, a lack of interest in activities, and general withdrawal. When depression predominates over psychotic symptoms, the diagnosis of schizoaffective disorder or even bipolar disorder might be considered.

14. Are memory problems symptoms of schizophrenia?

Schizophrenia is clearly distinguishable from Alzheimer's disease, where deficits in recent memory are prominent. A subtle cognitive disturbance, however, is clearly present in patients with schizophrenia at an early stage of illness. It is now known from some large research studies that IQ falls some time just before the onset of illness, and particularly that verbal memory and measures of learning that are called short-term "**working memory**" are often impaired throughout the illness, although most studies do not find that these deficits in **cognition** are progressive after the start of a full-blown illness. The greatest change in cognitive functioning and abilities seems to occur during the prodromal stage of the illness, i.e., in that 1- to 2-year period before those around the person with schizophrenia notice the signs of illness. Some of the cognitive changes may also stem from an early brain or adolescent developmental problem. The prodromal stage of schizophrenia varies considerable in length, with some patients never appearing cognitively normal from early childhood, while others do well until late adolescence and have more abrupt downhill course in functioning.

Working memory

This is a more contemporary term for short-term memory. It is thought of as an active system for temporarily storing and manipulating information needed for conducting complex tasks, such as learning, reasoning, and comprehending things.

Cognition

The quality of the mind that allows animals and humans to think, reason, and manipulate their environment to survive.

The underlying causes and mechanisms of the impairments are not known. For example, is there a memory information retrieval problem, as some studies seem to suggest, or an information storage problem? Sometimes the memory and learning problems are confused with an attention problem. Regardless, people with schizophrenia do not learn new things as well as people without schizophrenia, particularly things of a complex, sequential nature. It is assumed that the cognitive problems stem from structural (and thus functional) disturbances in the frontal and temporal cortices of the brain, particularly on the left side—the regions where language is processed. People who have relatively high cognitive functioning prior to a schizophrenia-like illness may not be impaired cognitively once they develop illness, and there is some thought that a high IQ may be somewhat protective from the severe consequences or outcomes for this illness.

Some medications that are used to treat the side effects of some of the older neuroleptic medications, such as benztropine (Cogentin®), can have an effect on memory, and this should be taken into account during evaluations of memory problems. If the patient is taken off this medication, memory may improve.

15. Do people with schizophrenia have a low IQ?

Most individuals with schizophrenia have normal intelligence; however, there is a drop in each individual's IQ at the beginning of illness (see Question 14). In contrast, however, some mental retardation syndromes (relatively low IQ) do co-occur with schizophrenia, and when present, this may give clues to the origin of the disorder in those individuals. Usually the latter cases have very poor premorbid histories, with the individuals having been educated in special classes in childhood and multiple therapeutic interventions before adolescence. They may have an underlying rare genetic disorder that could now be determined by **DNA** testing at any of the several commercial genetic testing companies.

DNA

DNA is made of different nucleic acids: adenine, guanine, thiamine, and cytosine and is put together in the form of a triple helical structure. The variation in genes between individuals depends on the sequence that these nucleic acids appear in an individual's genes.

16. *Are muscular problems associated with schizophrenia?*

It used to be thought that any motor problems present in people with schizophrenia, such as the well-known example of severe tardive dyskinesia, were a consequence of medications. It is now recognized, and was many decades ago, that some motor disturbances and strange movements known as **dyskinesias** are present in patients as they are becoming ill, before they start any medications. In fact, some studies show that motor development (age at first walking) is somewhat delayed during early childhood in people who later develop schizophrenia, and even at birth some abnormal, clumsy movements were detected by one investigator in some now-famous home movies. **Tardive dyskinesia**, which is a debilitating motor disturbance thought to occur after years of being administrated medications such as chlorpromazine (Thorazine), fluphenazine (Prolixin) and haloperidol (Haldol), is also known to occur in some patients who have never been on these medications.

Dyskinesia

Difficulty in performing movements voluntarily. See also **Tardive dyskinesia**.

Tardive dyskinesia

A debilitating motor disturbance consisting of pronounced, uncontrollable motor movements of the limbs and tongue that sometimes occurred as a side effect of older antipsychotic medications.

17. Do people with schizophrenia have a reduced life span or die from their illness?

It is doubtful that schizophrenia directly reduces one's life span. There are even debates as to whether incidences of certain cancers are more rare among people with schizophrenia than in the general population. If large populations are studied, however, the age at death is lower in people with schizophrenia because of their being increasingly prone to accidents, increased suicide rates, and in severe cases, chronic institutionalization, which may produce a lack of rigorous health care and proper nutrition, as well as acceleration of aging possibly because of the multiple combinations of medications with many adverse side effects that people with chronic schizophrenia tend to take for many years. Even today, people with schizophrenia tend not to obtain adequate health care and preventive dietary and health-related measures that can work toward increasing one's life span. There are also some healthcare professionals who may be biased against patients with a known chronic illness such as schizophrenia such that when patients with this disorder visit an emergency room for pain, the physician may quickly triage them to psychiatry services, overlooking an important medical diagnosis. This is a public health problem that needs to be addressed.

18. Are there medical conditions that look like schizophrenia?

Countless other illnesses are sometimes accompanied by hallucinations and delusions, from metabolic disturbances influencing the brain to viral illnesses, brain tumors, and specific chromosomal abnormalities. The specific aspect of the auditory hallucinations, however, might be different from what is generally seen in schizophrenia. For example, more than one voice talking about the subject or one voice commenting on the subject's actions is more specific to schizophrenia. The course of illness is more characteristic as well and can be an indication pointing to a schizophrenia diagnosis. All the other mentioned causes have other physical symptoms accompanying the psychosis that are uncharacteristic of schizophrenia.

When someone presents to a physician with what appears to be a first episode of schizophrenia, good medical practice dictates that these other conditions should be excluded, particularly if there is any indication that they might be present or the characteristics that are seen on the first episode are in any way atypical of schizophrenia. Some of the examples, both common and rare, of medical illnesses that can masquerade as schizophrenia are phenylketonuria, Huntington's disease, lupus erythematosus, thyroid disease, parathyroid disease, vitamin B12 deficinecy, and chronic alcohol and drug abuse. These are just a few examples of many that can be ruled out by testing and other diagnostic processes before a schizophrenia diagnosis is made.

19. Do people with schizophrenia have fewer offspring?

Fertility and **fecundity** are two different entities. People with schizophrenia, if withdrawn and behaviorally different, may not want mates and may not appear attractive to others. Their difficulties in forming close relations generalize to sexual problems as well. This is more true of males than of females, and thus, some studies show

Fertility
Having the normal biology that gives one the ability to bear children.

Fecundity
Bearing children.

that the number of offspring of males with schizophrenia is lower than that of females. It is thus thought to be a fecundity problem and not likely to be reduced fertility for biologic reasons. Some possible causes of schizophrenia, such as chromosomal microdeletions and chromosomal insertions, may also produce reduced fertility as a tertiary effect of the genetic defect, but this is not an outcome of the illness itself.

This may cause one to wonder why an illness that leads to reduced offspring is not decreasing in incidence. In some diseases that continue despite reduced or nonexistent fertility, a genetic advantage is associated with the disadvantageous illness (such as in the case of sickle-cell anemia, which offers protection from malaria even while producing significant disease). However, no such relationship has been described for schizophrenia. Alternatively, evidence from new genetic studies is also implicating spontaneous new gene mutations as a source of illness that could explain its continuation over time. Why schizophrenia still exists today and is not declining in incidence is still unclear; it may be due to more than one reason, and is an important question for researchers to further explore.

20. Do people diagnosed with a first episode of schizophrenia recover? If so, how long will this take?

A substantial number of patients recover fully from a first episode of schizophrenia within a couple of months after it is identified and treated, although the percentage of patients who are back to their premorbid state by

5 years after the first episode is quite low—only about 10%. There are certain factors that are predictive of good outcome, which include short duration of untreated illness prior to the first episode, having affective symptoms (i.e. depression), continuing neuroleptic medication consistently, and having the benefit of various psychosocial treatments once the acute symptoms have resided—that is, having a therapist whom the individual visits on a regular, frequent basis and having family support and understanding. Various approaches that supplement treatment, such a cognitive therapy, training to improve social skills, supportive housing, vocational training and placement, and family therapy and psycho-education can improve the chances of a good outcome.

There are several large studies worldwide that have examined populations of first-episode patients to determine what predicts good outcome and what interventions can be used to increase chances of a good outcome. In the United States, the National Institutes of Mental Health (NIMH) has been sponsoring a program called Recovery After an Initial Schizophrenia Episode (RAISE), a nationwide set of community-based programs that aggressively identify the illness early in its evolution and treat with the combined interventions described earlier. Each center is different in that the resources, financial base, and populations vary. However, results from all of them will ultimately be combined to offer clinicians a standard for how a first episode of psychotic illness should be approached.

21. What is the course of chronic schizophrenia over time, and what can influence it?

No clear predictors of illness course exist, and hopefully, more biological variables will be affirmed in the future. Females tend to have a milder course of illness and a later age of onset than males by about a mean of two years. Early age of onset and poor premorbid social and academic functioning, along with a long duration of untreated psychosis, are hallmarks of a more severe course of illness.

The old adage about schizophrenia is that one-third of first-episode cases of schizophrenia go on to a chronic deteriorating course, one-third are in the middle—patients who have the illness but can function (albeit at a lower level than previously)—and one-third never have another episode again. The latter statistic is now thought to be overly optimistic. Although many individuals do quite well, it is generally believed that no more than 10% of individuals who have a clear first episode of schizophrenia can consider themselves recovered afterward without medication (see above, and see **Part 2**, Questions 30–35). Many people may find that they essentially have no symptoms while on medication. Others may recover, only to relapse again as long as 5 years later.

Unfortunately, after recovery from the acute stages of a first episode, many patients think that they do not need medication, stop taking it, and eventually relapse. Additionally, the time to a second episode varies. Often it does not occur immediately, but may take a few years to again develop. Currently, with the advent of new medications that have almost no side effects, a stable dose can be achieved for a period of several years without the patient feeling the uncomfortable side effects of the old medications. The course of illness in the population as a whole may have changed and become milder as a result of early vigorous treatment with new medications and better compliance among patients. If left untreated, the natural course of schizophrenia is a lifetime of symptoms and deterioration.

Before the widespread use of neuroleptic medications, patients were hospitalized for years and lived the rest of their lives on the "back wards" of public hospitals, deteriorating in manner and cognition. It was hard to distinguish between this course of illness and the environmentally deprived effects of institutionalization. When government legislation for the establishment of community mental health centers came in vogue in the 1960s to 1970s, medicated patients were discharged from hospitals and returned to the community. The effects of long-term institutionalization were recognized, but not solved. Often, the living environments that patients were transferred to were in many ways impoverished and unsupportive to the needs of these individuals. As a consequence of this dreary and problematic environment—and partially the underlying illness itself—many patients returned frequently to the hospitals, and the so-called "revolving door" phenomenon began to take effect. Throughout their lifetime, patients began to have records filled with numerous admissions and discharges. State-allotted funds for the inpatient institutions have dwindled each year, resulting in at most only a few hundred beds per state hospital—or even none in states where state-run hospitals have closed. It is common to drive now through the grounds of the state facilities—once lively, self-sustaining communities in themselves—and see many buildings boarded up and vacant, with weeds growing on the once well-manicured grounds surrounding the buildings. Such closures might lead one to believe that serious mental illness is disappearing, but this is actually untrue. The incidence and prevalence of schizophrenia worldwide is the same as it has been for decades. What *has* changed is that we are tempering the course of the illness with new medications so that more patients are able to be cared for directly in the community, at least in the U.S. and other Western countries.

Currently, however, mental health care is in a crisis in the United States (as is health care in general). With serious mental illness, this is an international crisis, of the proportion of the AIDS, Ebola, or other infectious disease epidemics. However, schizophrenia is a lifetime disorder that can now be effectively treated and cared for, although legislation in each country needs to be in place that is sensitive to the needs of the individuals disabled by this disease, instead of stigmatizing them and ignoring their legitimate need for health care. Nevertheless, the history of substandard care for the mentally ill in the United States and other Western countries is hopefully part of the past. There is current optimism that if continually medicated, people with schizophrenia now can lead normal, productive lives and don't have to be burdened by uncomfortable symptoms or medication side effects.

22. What can patients and their families do to minimize symptoms and influence outcome?

Family members often ask what they can do to help their loved one to recover. Aside from seeing that the opportunities exist for the kinds of treatments and therapies mentioned above and encouraging the affected individual to seek them, compassion and understanding, and resisting the temptation to pressure him or her to "find a job or go back to school," are what is generally needed. Above all, keeping the individual safe from harming him or herself, recognizing the developing symptoms of a new episode, and helping the person organize his/her daily life is key. Joining support groups offered by organizations such as the National Alliance on Mental Illness (NAMI) and providing the opportunity for social networking at community centers can be helpful for the family and patient as well. Staying connected and knowing that others care and also experience the same phenomena can alleviate the "pain" of mental illness, and can dampen the pervasive suicidal thoughts that arise when someone is recovering from a first episode of psychosis.

23. What happens if someone opts for no treatment or gets the wrong treatment?

We do not know for sure what happens to people who are admitted to the hospital with a first psychotic episode and then deny they are ill and leave. As long as they are not disruptive in the community, they may go for years managing to survive either in their own home or on the streets. We do know, though, that they are highly unlikely to be living up to their full potential as one may have predicted from the state they were in prior to illness.

Can they get "the wrong treatment"? Certainly; however, what "wrong" might consist of varies. There are some groups who advocate against **antipsychotic** medication

Antipsychotic
Any medication that specifically suppresses the positive symptoms of hallucinations and delusions. This medication can also be useful in other conditions as a strong tranquilizer.

and psychiatrists. They have been less prevalent over the last couple of decades, particularly as educational support groups such as NAMI have sprung into existence, but nevertheless, these still exist, and we can only hope that individuals who take their recommendations eventually trust a clinician or community worker to guide them into the more widely recommended, effective treatments, such as those outlined in this book.

24. Are there some societies in which no individuals develop schizophrenia?

This is an interesting academic issue. E. Fuller Torrey (1980), in his book *Schizophrenia and Civilization*, described pockets of schizophrenia throughout the world and noted some isolated areas where it is nonexistent. He particularly described the highlands of Papua New Guinea as one region without evidence of schizophrenia. Currently, however, psychiatrists now practicing in Papua New Guinea say that Torrey certainly missed some cases, and documents of such cases in that region do exist in the literature. It would be interesting to study these societies closer. For example, the San tribes of South Africa are said to be the oldest African group in existence; they have isolated themselves from society, maintaining their prehistoric hunter–gatherer culture despite the surrounding civilization. Although there is some indication that schizophrenia does exist among these people, because of tribal laws, it has been difficult for Western-trained professionals to enter their communities to examine whether mental illness exists within the context of their culture.

Despite these rare mentioned examples, the World Health Organization has conducted studies over the years to show that schizophrenia is a disease of humanity and is universal. This fact alone may give clues to its genetic origin. For a genetic disorder to be universal, one possibility is that it may be as old as modern humans themselves. Modern ***Homo sapiens*** were derived from one genetic bottleneck formed in Africa approximately 150,000 years ago. However, one new gene mutation occuring at that time would be very unlikely to cause schizophrenia. One theory is that, since the capacity for complex language is distinctly human and schizophrenia can be seen as a disorder of the biologic pathways for language, genes that define the human capacity for language may somehow be related to schizophrenia. An alternative genetic explanation may be that spontaneous mutations (those that occur in the egg or sperm without having been present in the parent) frequently occur in specific genes, and one or more of these mutations may continue to lead to greater risk for schizophrenia.

Homo sapiens

The scientific designation for modern human beings.

PART 2

Treatment: When, Where, by Whom, and With What?

"The physician should not treat the disease but the patient who is suffering from it."

—Maimonides

Who first sees an individual with schizophrenia and what type of professional can treat the first symptoms

Why won't some psychiatrists treat people with schizophrenia?

What if I do not have insurance or my policy does not cover psychiatric care?

More . . .

25. Who first sees an individual with schizophrenia, and what type of professional can treat the first symptoms?

Many types of doctors and therapists are currently treating the first symptoms of schizophrenia, and because of the types of health services in the United States and other similar countries, the primary care practitioner (MD, DO, or NP), family physician, pediatrician, or emergency room doctor will likely be the first to treat the symptoms. However, even sooner, it is friends and family, a schoolteacher, nurse, or psychologist who may see the first evidence that illness is evolving, and yet not know what to do. Since the early warning signs can sometimes be indistinguishable from adolescent mood changes, general practitioners and pediatricians will often suggest that patients will "grow out of it," and that parental support and guidance are what is necessary. They tend to be reluctant to make a schizophrenia diagnosis given the stigma it produces (see Question 97).

Many cases have been made public of severely disturbed adolescents whose families and healthcare professionals, initially aware of their behavior, did not understand that an impending psychosis could be approaching. The 1999 Columbine High School murders in Colorado were certainly an example. The parents and teachers seemed largely unaware that delusional and bizarre changes were taking place in the boys, who had paired together out of common, extreme thoughts and interests. They were saying things and acting in a manner that those around them should have been able to detect as serious pathology that was brewing. Instead, they had been in a juvenile detention program and actually had social workers, who did not notice their downward spiraling.

Several more such incidences of early psychosis-related violence have since been reported in the news. The 2011 Tucson shooting of 18 people, including a well-known congresswoman, by a 22-year-old man is another example. He had previously been suspended from his college for bizarre and disruptive behavior, and his only prior bout with the law was an arrest on a minor drug charge. In 2012, a lone gunman shot and killed several people in an Aurora, Colorado movie theatre. Yet this young man, with a degree in neuroscience and pursuing a PhD program at the University of Colorado, had never been known to be violent, although he was in treatment for psychiatric symptoms and had been noted to be acting more troubled and bizarre just prior to the shootings. In the same year, a gunman stormed into a Newtown, Connecticut elementary school, killing several children and teachers. Another famous occurrence, the Long Island Railroad Massacre, was caused by a young adult who for several months became increasingly paranoid and delusional, but his symptoms remained unrecognized by all around him until he boarded a commuter train one evening from Penn Station, New York, with a rifle and shot several passengers randomly. There are several other such events worldwide that frequently, but not always, involve someone with an untreated, evolving schizophrenia-like illness. Of course, violent acts are certainly committed by people who do not have schizophrenia, and rather have a disdain and lack of respect for human life, with no ability for empathy or attachment; such people are often referred to as "sociopaths" or "antisocial" individuals. However, when they do involve someone who is developing schizophrenia and not yet being treated for this illness, it is due to the lack of proper identification of those first symptoms of schizophrenia, before they become a devastating crisis and harmful to other people or themselves. Although cases do not all culminate in a violent act before being recognized, these are extreme examples of what can happen when subtle signs are ignored by even people close to the person who is becoming ill. Better education of those first people to be in contact with these individuals might help to prevent such future episodes described here. (Violent behavior in schizophrenia is discussed further in **Part 7**.)

Although general, nonpsychiatric doctors may end up treating people with early schizophrenia, the best treatment will certainly be from trained psychiatrists who are versed in the early signs and latest medications, their optimal doses, efficacy, and side effects, as well as when and how long to medicate. In addition, specifically trained psychiatrists are knowledgeable about providing the needed follow-up and long-term care. This is, of course, the ideal situation, recognizing that many people with schizophrenia in the United States may quickly use up their health insurance benefits, or may not be covered at all and may lack the financial capacity to afford treatment. The medications are expensive, as is the continued care, and people with schizophrenia tend to be unable to obtain high-paying employment or maintain regular jobs with benefits. In fact, during the prodromal stage, which often lasts a couple of years, it is not uncommon for an individual to lose a job or drop out of college and thus forfeit medical insurance benefits. In countries where health care is available regardless of ability to pay, there still are long waits to receive the needed care, and the individual with schizophrenia is likely to be delusional and disorganized, and therefore unable to understand how to obtain the needed care, or even be unaware that it is needed. The latter is why an advocate for this individual's care is so important.

Pharmacotherapy is the primary treatment modality and is only prescribed through a medical doctor or license nurse practitioner. Although other therapies given by social workers or psychologists can help, such as supportive psychotherapy, **cognitive behavioral therapy (CBT)** (see Question 39), family therapy, and orthomolecular therapy (vitamin and mineral treatments), they must be used in conjunction with pharmacotherapy in order to relieve the major core symptoms. The other modalities are only supplements to medication and may facilitate and augment their effects, but do not replace them. The nonpharmacologic therapies may also help in daily functioning in a way that medication alone cannot. Pharmacotherapy certainly does not have all the answers; for example, some patients do not respond well to medications and may even have uncomfortable side effects. Medications do not yet "cure" the actual biological basis for the illness but are likely to be effective for suppressing the symptoms, much like aspirin suppresses the fever and headache from influenza without actually resolving the infection.

Pharmacotherapy

Treatment with prescription medications under the supervision of a physician.

Cognitive behavioral therapy (CBT)

This is a brief form of psychotherapy based on the principle that the way one thinks about something causes actions. Thus, it is focused on changing thinking patterns that lead to disruptive behavior.

After a patient is stabilized on medication, the psychotherapist, social workers, and occupational therapists need to take a role in providing the social treatments that are needed to improve the quality of life of people with schizophrenia. Rarely will a psychiatrist, who has many patients on his or her roster, have or take the time to follow up on a patient's practical needs or to make sure that the patient complies with the proper medication regime and other services. The role of other professionals is essential for the support necessary to achieve a favorable outcome for the illness of each patient (see, for instance, Question 20's discussion of the RAISE project).

26. Why won't some psychiatrists treat people with schizophrenia?

The average clinical psychiatrist in private practice frequently will decline to treat people with schizophrenia, at least in the United States, for several reasons. The first is that doctors fear liability from lawsuits if the patient does something harmful to himself/herself or others. These clinicians also fear the possibility of violence and aggression toward themselves, especially if they practice in isolated, private office settings. The second is that people with schizophrenia have limited resources and are almost always unemployed on a regular basis. The nature of their illness means that they will have difficulty working and have no insurance coverage. Even when patients come from families with considerable financial security, they can quickly drain parental savings. Psychiatrists in private practice can rarely see patients with schizophrenia and maintain a livelihood. Thus, these patients are generally seen only once every 3 to 4 months in clinics by physicians/psychiatrists and/or nurse practitioners who have large caseloads and are then followed up by caseworkers and psychiatric social workers more frequently.

Unfortunately, many people with schizophrenia never make it into a stable treatment setting and are lost to follow-up either after hospitalizations for acute episodes or because they leave the security of a parental home with support and wander away aimlessly, sometimes living on the street as a result of the symptoms.

27. What if I do not have insurance or my policy does not cover psychiatric care?

Although a lack of insurance is clearly a serious problem with health care today in the United States and some other countries, the current system is not hopeless. The Patient Protection and Affordable Care Act (also called the ACA or "Obamacare") in the U.S. has extended insurance coverage to many more people and families in the last couple of years. The Affordable Care Act provides further help for families because they may now keep children on health insurance policies until age 26, which helps at least with the first few years of illness. Where it fails, however, is in the ability of parents to provide long-term care for their adult children with schizophrenia.

Some public hospital emergency rooms will provide acute care and then make referrals to an appropriate clinic. If the individual served in the U.S. armed forces, he/she is also entitled to coverage within the Veterans Administration's healthcare system. The social worker assigned to an emergency room often knows what is available in your area. In addition, there are sliding pay scales and many kind-hearted psychiatrists who will allow the patient to pay only what he or she can afford. Each state has its own system for public care of the mentally ill and most patients take advantage of their state systems, since no one is turned away for lack of funds.

The U.S. federal government has passed legislation for "parity in health care" for mental illness. Legislatures recognized that schizophrenia and other psychiatric disorders are medical illnesses that warrant coverage that is equal to diabetes, hypertension, and other chronic illnesses. This has taken a lot of public education, and it has been difficult to get Congress to bring such a bill onto the floor of the House and Senate. Sponsored by Senators Paul Wellstone and Pete Domenici, the Mental Health Parity and Addiction Equity Act amends the *Employee Retirement Income Security Act* and the Public Health Service Act to prohibit employers' health plans from imposing any caps or limitations on mental health treatment or substance use disorder benefits that aren't applied to medical and surgical benefits. The Mental Health Parity and Addiction Equity Act does not require health insurance plans to provide mental health or substance use disorder benefits. However, for group health plans with 50 or more employees that choose to provide mental health and substance use disorder benefits, the Act does require parity with medical and surgical benefits. Thus, group health plans that provide both medical and surgical benefits and mental health and substance use disorder benefits may not impose financial requirements and treatment limitations applicable to mental health and substance use disorder benefits that are more restrictive than the financial requirements and treatment limitations applied to medical and surgical benefits. Requirements such as co-payments and deductibles and limitations such as number of visits or frequency of treatments can be no more restrictive on mental health and substance use disorder benefits than the requirements or limitations imposed on medical and surgical benefits. However, this law in no way requires that insurance plans provide coverage for treatment of mental illness, only that when services are covered, they must be equal to medical and surgical benefits.

Another way to find appropriate healthcare services is to find the nearest local National Alliance for the Mentally Ill (NAMI) chapter. NAMI will have knowledge of the best places to go for immediate treatment and will be able to give advice based on experience often with their own family members. They serve not only as a resource in difficult times but as important continued support for people dealing with mental illness in their families.

These answers are all very specific to health care in the United States. The availability and parity for treatment of mental illness varies considerably worldwide and depends on the type of healthcare payment system for each individual country and the availability of different healthcare professionals to provide the services needed.

28. Do I have to be treated in a hospital if I have schizophrenia? If so, for how long?

Often, unfortunately, the first time that someone's symptoms of schizophrenia are noticed is when he or she is psychotic (lacking awareness of reality to the point that he/she could be harmful to themselves or others). In this case, patients rarely volunteer to go to a hospital and are either forcefully brought there by family or friends, or picked up by the police. In some countries, crisis teams may be available to make home visits and determine the urgency for immediate treatment, providing the transportation as needed. In many countries, particularly in impoverished nations, progress in modernizing hospitals is far behind the Western world, and the reputation of psychiatric hospitals is such that after someone is placed there, he or she is thought to "disappear" and not come back. There is thus a terrible fear of psychiatric institutions. Often the hospitals are so ill-equipped and poorly staffed that they become more of a way to isolate people from society rather than a facility for humanely treating patients with the latest medications. Such was the case when I went to visit the National Psychiatric Hospital in El Salvador. It surprised me that even the library, where psychiatrists should be able to get the latest advice, had no major journals. Only outdated copies of *The American Journal of Psychiatry* from 10 years prior to my visit were on the shelves. In other countries, such as within central Africa, relatives keep afflicted individuals locked in chains to walls or doorknobs of homes in order to keep them from harming themselves or other people.

Much publicity occurred many years ago about the conditions of psychiatric hospitals in the United States, which provided the material for Hollywood movies such as *The Snake Pit*, which I saw as a child, or *One Flew over the Cuckoo's Nest* from the 1960s. Even a more recent movie, *Changeling* with Angelina Jolie, invokes images of psychiatric hospitals that have long been forgotten in the United States—but not necessarily worldwide.

Truthfully, many years ago lobotomies were practiced as *One Flew over the Cuckoo's Nest* depicts, and patients lived in squalor as in *The Snake Pit*. However, these practices have clearly changed. Most general hospitals in the United States and other industrialized nations have psychiatry wards, and patients with schizophrenia are kept only as long as required to be stabilized on medication (usually 10 to 30 days) before being transferred into appropriate, longer-term outpatient treatment. Mainly, it is required when it is necessary to keep the patient safe from harming him or herself or others. When this is no longer needed, the patient can be released. Often hospitalization is best for the patient once medications are initiated because, not only can the patient be under close observation for side effects, but also it takes time for the medications to work and during that period, the illness could escalate.

Nevertheless, despite the "modernization" of psychiatric hospitals and wards, the atmosphere on the typical unit is still very different from hospital medical wards. Patients usually do not have private rooms; there is generally a large day room where patients can sit, watch TV, play games; there can be a room for sitting with outside visitors, but wards are locked, and individual sleeping rooms do not have private bathrooms, telephones, or TVs. When someone is hospitalized for the first time, they can feel overwhelmed quickly by this atmosphere and the other, very ill patients around them. The staff working with the patient are all sensitive to these issues and attempt in helping him/her adjust, but it can be a difficult time.

29. What treatments were used before pharmaceutical companies introduced neuroleptic medication?

The history of pharmacologic treatment for schizophrenia is interesting and is available in several very readable classic articles (e.g., Lehmann and Ban, 1997) and books (Fink, 1999; Whitaker, 2002), although many espouse the authors' prejudices against psychiatry more than relay the facts. The 2005 best-selling novel in the United Kingdom, *Human Traces* by Sebastian Faulks, gives an interesting historical account of the treatment of people with mental illness over a century ago, but unfortunately, this book strays somewhat from the truth when it endows its psychiatrists with the creative hypotheses about the uniquely human nature of schizophrenia that was coincidentally suggested by a more contemporary psychiatric researcher, Professor Timothy Crow of Oxford, nearly a century later (Crow, 1997).

People with the symptoms of schizophrenia have always stood out as not belonging in society because of the extreme oddness in the way they look or act. Thus, they have often been dubbed with the terms of "crazy," "loco," "mad," etc. During the late 1800s to the early 20th century and even before, there was a big movement in the U.S. and Europe to create large psychiatric institutions to house these individuals and place them far from urban areas. This focus on the question of management of the mentally ill led some to believe that schizophrenia was actually increasing in epidemic proportions throughout Western civilization (Torrey and Miller, 2000), although most researchers believe that this idea has no scientific basis, but rather is due to changes in diagnostic systems and definitions of **insanity**.

Insanity
Mental malfunctioning or unsoundness of mind to produce lack of judgment to the degree that the individual cannot determine right from wrong. The word tends to be used in a legal context rather than a medical one.

Lobotomy
The surgical division of one or more brain tracts. It is usually referred to as cutting a nerve that runs from the frontal lobe to the thalamus in the brain. It has been done in various ways, most often by inserting a needle above the nose in-between the eyes. This serves to disconnect nerves connecting the frontal lobe of the brain to other structures.

In the early part of the 20th century, Egas Moniz in Portugal developed a new technique (for which he received the Nobel Prize in Medicine) called "leukotomy." This surgical procedure involved drilling holes in the skull above the temporal lobes and then with the use of a needle-like instrument disrupting connections in brain tissue from several regions of the frontal lobes. This procedure was reported to alleviate the anxiety, agitation, and uncontrollable psychological stress of severely ill, institutionalized mental patients. Shortly afterward, Freedman adopted this technique in the United States and performed a few thousand leukotomies (renamed "**lobotomy**") in many patients during the peak of its popularity in the mid 1900s (El-Hai, 2005).

From the late 1930s through the 1950s, lobotomies were widely accepted as good practice in psychiatry throughout the mental hospitals in the United States. Although some individuals were dramatically helped by this procedure, there was also much abuse of its use, extending the indications for lobotomies to patients whom the nursing staff simply found "difficult" and whose behavioral problems disrupted the social setting of institutional life. Even the very wealthy and well-connected families (as in the famous case of Joseph and Rose Kennedy's daughter, Rosemary) had lobotomies performed unscrupulously on affected family members. There are still some parts of the world, such as countries of South America, where lobotomies are being performed on some patients, although this practice long ago disappeared in the U.S. and most Westernized countries.

Much of the treatment used during these times was primarily focused on isolating the ill person from society. Various therapies without proven scientific merit were given, including packing the patient in ice, bloodletting, prolonged sleep therapy, fever induction, and even tooth removal. Insulin shock therapy, in which patients were injected with large doses of insulin over several weeks to send them into daily comas, was a popular treatment in the mid 20th century. Behavior was contained by restraints and chaining. Most hospital wards not only had baths for placing people in cold-packs through a great part of the 20th century, but also had several isolation rooms so that agitated patients could be taken away from the rest of the patients and staff. Often, patients were in these rooms for longer than necessary because of the staff's fear. On some rare occasions, patients who may have been misdiagnosed and were withdrawing from addictive drugs or had cardiac problems unfortunately died while in this kind of therapy. While acute psychiatric wards still make use of seclusion rooms and leather restraints for patients in a very agitated, out-of-control and dangerous state today, strict guidelines for their use include careful monitoring and removing the patients within a few hours are now standard, unlike the practices of many years ago.

By the mid 20th century, psychoanalysis for schizophrenia became popular and was practiced well into the 1970s in some famous institutions for the well-to-do, such as the Menninger Clinic in Kansas and Chestnut Lodge in Maryland. Chestnut Lodge, a beautifully situated campus with lavish rooms and dining facilities and a lovely swimming pool for patient exercise, exposed people to the therapies developed by the well-known analyst Frieda Fromm-Reichman and became popularized by the novel *I Never Promised You a Rose Garden*. Patients were said to need psychoanalytic regression back to infancy and then mothering again through the stages of development slowly for symptomatic improvement and regaining a proper sense of reality. In the 1980s, Chestnut Lodge was threatened with losing its accreditation unless neuroleptics were reinstated in the treatment regime for all patients with schizophrenia, and thus, the institution gradually lost the attraction it once had for wealthy families of affected individuals. It fell into disrepute and eventually closed. Nevertheless, there are still such exclusive private institutions that can be found such as this that emphasize psychoanalysis and related therapies, but do prescribe medications as needed as well.

30. What are the current choices for medication?

In the modern era, it is generally believed by psychiatrists that there are no viable alternatives to medications, and advertisements for so-called "non-neuroleptic alternatives" are misleading. Some of these "alternative therapies," such as vitamins and dietary supplements, have no effect; others may have some modest effect or have an effect on specific symptoms, such as transcranial magnetic stimulation (TMS). Supportive psychotherapy and forms of cognitive therapies and family therapy are all adjunctive treatment to medications.

In 1952, Delay, Deniker and Harl were the first to report the antipsychotic effects of chlorpromazine, a compound developed to provide a sedative anesthesia for the French surgeon, Laborit. During the 1960s, large treatment trials, particularly in the U.S., established **phenothiazines** as the mainstay treatment for schizophrenia (chlorpromazine, called Thorazine as its trade name, being the prototype). It is now recognized from analysis of those treatment trials that the outcome is better if individuals with schizophrenia receive this treatment early in the course of the illness. In fact, it has been said that the new medications "emptied" the psychiatric hospitals of the long-term patients in the 1960s and brought people with schizophrenia into the mainstream of society. Severe, variable side effects of these medications still existed, however, and doses went higher and higher to achieve optimal clinical effects. Many patients still did not respond even to very high doses. Many other compounds of this class of drugs in addition to chlorpromazine were introduced by different pharmaceutical companies (e.g., perphenazine, trifluoperazine, and fluphenazine). Many of the phenothiazines were only known to patients by their tradenames, but these are rarely in use today: Thorazine, Mellaril, trilafon, Stelazine, and, Prolixin) While they had the same overall effects on suppressing the positive symptoms of schizophrenia (hallucinations and delusions), their side effects varied by having different relative chances of each for producing sedation, hypotension, stiffness, and lowering the seizure threshold. In fact, patients placed on these drugs had a certain appearance that could be quickly detected by the public as a stiff, staring demeanor that contributed to the stigmatization of people with serious mental illness.

Phenothiazines
A class of antipsychotic medications developed in the mid-20th century that proved useful in treating schizophrenia.

During this same time, in the 1950s, another class of drug, reserpine, derived from the plants of the genus *Rauvolfia*, was given for schizophrenia with some success, and was used frequently until phenothiazines became widespread. Similarly, about the same time in the late 1950s, haloperidol was developed by Paul Janssen in his laboratories in Belgium, and was also a byproduct of an analgesic used in anesthesia, but known to have the same behavioral properties as the phenothiazines and yet more potent. Haloperidol was introduced in the U.S. in 1967. Shortly afterwards, drugs with similar clinical and receptor profiles but different chemical structures were developed, namely flupenthixole, thiothixine (Navane), pimozide, loxapine (Loxitane), and molindone (Moban). All these first-generation drugs were thought to exert their action predominantly by blocking one of the receptors for a major brain chemical transmitter, **dopamine** (labeled the "D-2 receptor"), but had actions on other receptors as well and were not considered "clean drugs" chemically.

Dopamine

A neurotransmitter that is important for conveying "messages" between nerve cells in the brain.

In the 1970s, clozapine was introduced in Europe. This was a drug that had remarkable effects in patients who did not respond to the usual medications. It was thought to have a greater effect on receptors for serotonin, another one of the important brain transmitters, and thus has a very different receptor profile than the first-generation drugs. Initially, clozapine was not introduced in the U.S. because of its propensity to cause hypotension and thus dizziness, as well as seizures. Then when cases were reported of life-threatening leukopenia caused by clozapine, causing death in some patients in rare instances, its use was limited and it was not placed on the market in the United States. By the late 1980s, however, there was renewed interest in clozapine in the United States, and reports were making the newspapers of miraculous recoveries of individuals who had been completely psychotic and thought-disordered before clozapine, but then reverted to normal behavior, were released from the hospital, and applied for employment while taking this new drug. They also, most importantly, did not have the "look" that stigmatized so many patients taking the first-generation drugs. It was later noted that clozapine seemed to have a unique effect on preventing suicidal tendencies in patients with schizophrenia.

As a result of these findings from treatment trials using clozapine, the FDA approved its use for treatment of patients with tardive dyskinesia in 1989, as it appeared not to lead to this serious side effect. It was also approved for patients who were nonresponsive to trials of at least two other medications. The disadvantage to the patient is that he/she needs to be monitored closely with blood testing on a frequent basis to assure that blood dyscrasias, such as the leukopenia seen in the past, do not develop. The disadvantage to the psychiatrist using this drug is that he/she must first register the patient in a national registry and comply with the rules of the registry for use of this drug (see below). Thus, there is extra "red tape" in prescribing this medication, and many practitioners shy away from its use and are reluctant to place patients on clozapine, even when they or their caregivers request it. However, its value today as a primary treatment for schizophrenia should not be overlooked. No cases of serious leukopenia or deaths have been reported since its reinstitution. It does still have a black-box warning for agranulocytosis, seizures, myocarditis, and other cardiovascular and respiratory effects. It also is known to be more toxic in the elderly, particularly those with dementia, and could cause a delirium-like state.

Beginning in the early 1990s, many pharmaceutical companies began announcing the development of other new drugs for schizophrenia that have neurochemical mechanisms that are similar, although not identical, to clozapine, but that are less toxic to the blood system. Several of these have now reached the market and have been used for the last two decades or more. They have been dubbed the second-generation neuroleptics, or "atypicals," and include the drugs risperidone (Risperdal), olanzapine (Zyprexa), quetiapine (Seroquel), aripiprazole (Abilify), and ziprasidone (Geodon), and more recently the drug lurasidone (Latuda). These drugs may go by different trade names in other countries, but are produced by the global offices of all the major companies. Doses and potency vary among these drugs, but in general they have the same efficacy, much lower incidence of side effects, and thus good tolerability compared with the earlier generation of drugs such as haloperidol, chlorpromazine, thioridazine, perphenazine, thiothixine, and others.

While there is a lower incidence of side effects, they do still occur. For example, people taking risperidone have been known to complain of dizziness when standing (called "orthostatic hypotension") or may have their blood pressure go down too low. Males taking it may also, on rare occasions, suffer from gynecomastia (breast enlargement) and women from breast milk secretion. Many patients also do not like taking olanzapine and quetiapine because they then suffer from uncomfortable weight gain and are more prone to diabetes.

Many chronic patients are still medicated with first-generation drugs. They are much less expensive, as the drug companies no longer hold patents on them, and their efficacy is really not any different than the atypicals, as has been shown in some recent large treatment trials. The price differential, however, may shortly change as the second-generation drugs also come off patent. Regardless of the inconveniences, in clinical practice, if a patient doesn't respond to a typical or an atypical drug and has not yet been given a trial of clozapine, they should be started on it because the incidence of response to clozapine in patients nonresponsive to other drugs is still greater than with any of the other above-mentioned drugs. Sometimes in the very difficult and nonresponsive patient, a combination of clozapine and a drug such as risperidone is helpful, as the synergism between them allows for all the needed receptor blockade to occur and the risperidone tends to raise the blood levels of clozapine. (More discussion of combinations of drugs is in Question 31.)

31. Are combinations of different medications more effective than one alone?

Reality is that there appears to be a huge gap between research and clinical practice. Researchers tend to frown on so-called **polypharmacy**—giving combinations of different drugs having the same actions—and in support of their view cite the fact that there are no good double-blind controlled trials to support it. They recommend using only one drug at a time, and if it is not effective, tapering the patient off that drug and trying another. However, polypharmacy appears to be by far the most common practice of the majority of clinical psychiatrists who provide care to chronic patients with schizophrenia. The problem psychiatrists face is that they will often have a patient who is not responding sufficiently to one medication, but that medication is felt to at least keep the patient stable and out of the hospital. Thus, it is

Polypharmacy

The use of combinations of drugs to address the same problem or illness.

Decompensate

To deteriorate into a less functional state.

too risky to withdraw that medication and substitute another that will have unknown benefits for that patient and may make the patient **decompensate**, or deteriorate into a less functional state. The result is that the psychiatrist will choose instead to add the second drug onto the first. The difficulty with this situation is that if the patient improves, it cannot be determined whether the second drug is having the effect by itself or if the combination of the two is what is making the difference. If this patient then is seen by a new psychiatrist, that provider will be unwilling to change the medications if the patient is stable; thus, the patient is treated with polypharmacy even if it is uncertain whether it is necessary. Frequently, patients are found to be administered both typical and atypical neuroleptics combined with an added mood-stabilizing drug (valproic acid, carbamazepine, or lamotrigine) to "calm" them. These drugs appear to take away agitation and irritability and thus are called "mood stabilizers"; they are therapeutic for seizure disorders, but also have been used for mania. Based on unmet clinical needs and modest evidence from case reports, combinations of two or more second-generation drugs may merit future investigation in efficacy trials involving patients with schizophrenia who have treatment-resistant illness (including partial response) or who are responsive to treatment but develop intolerable adverse effects and so are prescribed subtherapeutic doses of each drug which, when combined, may alleviate symptoms. Other situations that may merit polypharmacy are when schizophrenia is accompanied by comorbid conditions (e.g., anxiety, depression, suicidal or self-injurious behavior, aggression). In certain clinical situations, combining a drug for schizophrenia with an antidepressent, moodstabilizer, or antianxiety medication may be superior to monotherapy. However, the research data thus far is not clear about this.

32. When to use clozapine and if it doesn't work, then what?

Clozapine is currently the most efficacious antipsychotic medication available to patients with schizophrenia. However, because of its side effects, it's not the first treatment of choice during a first psychotic episode. It should, however, be considered if someone has been given a trial of at least two different antipsychotics, preferably risperidone, olanzapine, and/or perphenazine, for at least a month each without much response in terms of disappearance of the positive symptoms, i.e., hallucinations, disordered speech, and delusions. The dose of these medications should have been in the therapeutic range, and the patient should have been consistently taking them as prescribed; if these criteria are met and the patient still doesn't respond, then a trial of clozapine may be warranted. Until the patient is stable, not only should a blood sample be drawn once a week to make sure the more serious side effects of leukopenia (reduced white blood cell count) and specifically neutropenia can be detected early, but also a clozapine blood level is helpful to determine whether the dose is producing a level in the blood that is known to be therapeutic, as the dose that can be effective ranges from 100 mg to a little over 400 mg daily.

Clozapine treatment is usually begun slowly, titrating up to the correct blood level in increments of 25 mg every few days or a week at a time. Once a dose of about 100 mg is achieved, some response may be seen, but usually a dose of between 300–400 mg is necessary to achieve a high enough blood level for significant response.

In general, a patient is considered to have had an adequate trial of the drug if the blood level is reported to be above 400 ng/ml. The minor side effects, which may subside over time if a patient can tolerate them, are generally a lowering of blood pressure, dizziness on standing, sleepiness, and drooling, the latter of which is probably the most bothersome to patients. The daily dose can all be given at bedtime, to minimize the intolerability of side effects. Absorption varies among individuals, and thus it is important to know whether a therapeutic blood level has been reached. Other side effects are rare, but have been reported. These vary in seriousness and include risk of seizures, myocarditis, or psychotic dementia or sudden death occurring in elderly patients treated with this drug. It can also increase the risk for diabetes and raise blood glucose (sugar) values.

A prescriber of clozapine in the U.S. must register him/herself and the patient in a clozapine National Registry (www.clozapineregistry.com) as mandated by the FDA. Pharmacies dispensing clozapine must also be registered. All drug companies that manufacture clozapine have their own registries. The registries will hopefully prevent challenging of patients with clozapine who have already had serious reduction of white blood cell counts should they go for treatment in a facility that does not know the patient's history, as patients are often not good historians about these events. White blood cell and absolute neutrophil counts (ANCs) are monitored weekly and reported to the national center. Of course, if an emergency exists and the patient cannot obtain a blood draw at exactly a week's time, then a 1-week emergency prescription is allowable. Pharmacies carefully regulate the distribution of this drug such that patients can only receive refills when their blood has been checked and acceptable results confirmed on a weekly basis. It is likely for this reason that consumers find that many doctors will not prescribe clozapine for patients. The added government control takes extra time that is often not available in busy practices or clinics.

33. Are there any new possibilities for treatments on the horizon?

Several of the drug companies are currently in the early stages of developing new classes of drugs for schizophrenia. While several recent trials of drugs targeting the glutamatergic neurotransmitter system have not shown efficacy (the exception being ketamine trials for depressive symptoms), others are being developed that have anti-inflammatory efficacy, based on new evidence that inflammation in the brain could be occurring early on in the illness. Some drugs that slow the general neurodegeneration of the aging process (so-called "oxidative stress") are also being sought. Finally, another area of interest appears to be hormonal. For example, **oxytocin**, the hormone released by the pituitary gland during labor and involved in sexual behaviors, is also a neuromodulator and has been shown to be useful in treating some of the symptoms of schizophrenia. Even estrogen receptor modulators, such as raloxifene (Evista), currently used to prevent breast cancer in at-risk women, are currently in treatment trials and may hold some efficacy for specific symptoms of schizophrenia.

Oxytocin
A neuromodulating hormone useful in treating some schizophrenia symptoms.

As discussed in Question 20, NIMH has funded a large clinical research initiative aimed at determining the most optimal path for treatment of a first episode of schizophrenia in a "real-world" clinical setting to improve the functional outcome of patients. This project, called RAISE (Recovery After an Initial Schizophrenia Episode) involved multiple clinical settings throughout the United States and has developed a combined pharmacologic and psychosocial treatment regime with a training module that is hoped to improve outcome and provide an elevated standard of care early on in the illness that will ultimately have an impact on the course of illness for people with this disorder. Other, similar multicenter collaborative efforts have also been undertaken in European countries.

34. What are the medication side effects and how are they resolved?

Some of the side effects have been listed previously. The two side effects of the atypicals that have received a lot of publicity are substantial weight gain, more so with olanzapine than with the other drugs, and diabetes-like problems with glucose metabolism. Although each drug company will report studies indicating that their drug has fewer side effects than those of their competitors, and in many areas more efficacy, it is hard to tease out the bias in this reporting. Thus, the NIMH invested funds in a large, multicenter comparison trial called the Clinical Antipsychotic Trials of Intervention Effectiveness (CATIE) using several of these drugs and one of the older drugs as well to compare their efficacy and side effects. Surprisingly, few differences between the drugs have emerged. The older drugs, such as haloperidol, chlorpromazine, perphenazine and others, have not been used much in the United States over the past few years because the efficacy of the atypicals has been clearly proven and drug companies tend to push those medications that are still on patent (i.e., the newer atypicals). However, some other countries still predominantly use the older drugs, and thus, motor side effects are still common in patients from those countries. These drugs have also been shown to have metabolic side effects that are seen in the newer atypicals. Yet there is still clearly a role for these drugs in the management of schizophrenia in the Western world as well.

Mainly, the old medications produced grossly obvious Parkinsonian-like side effects (tremors and stiffness), and in some cases, tardive dyskinesia, a particularly severe side effect of pronounced, uncontrollable motor movements of the limbs and tongue. With the discontinuation of medication, sometimes it was reversible, but often not. Also, trials of discontinuation and then reinstitution of the medications often made tardive dyskinesia even worse. This debilitating condition was widely feared, not only because of the disability it caused but also because of the peculiar look it gave its victims, forcing them to stand out in public and be stigmatized even more so than from the stiffness and Parkinsonian symptoms mentioned above. Other side effects included sedation, dizziness, hypotension, a lack of sexual drive, and liver damage. These side effects appear less of a concern for the newer second-generation antipsychotics, although the metabolic syndrome (see **Box**, "What is Metabolic Syndrome?" on page 78) certainly continues to be a problem.

With respect to results of the CATIE study, clozapine was found to be the most efficacious, but for those patients who preferred not to take clozapine, olanzapine and risperidone seemed more effective than ziprasidone and quetiapine. But side effects varied within this group: Olanzapine was associated with substantial weight gain and metabolic problems, more so than the other medications; ziprasidone was consistently associated with reduction in weight and improvement in metabolic indicators. Risperidone showed the lowest rate of intolerable side effects.

One rare side effect is known as Neuroleptic Malignant Syndrome. This is a condition that usually develops after a person has been treated with neuroleptics in increasing doses because of lack of the first generation response. Instead of getting better, the patient appears worse and so even more medications are given at high doses. The hallmark signs of **neuroleptic malignant syndrome** (**NMS**) are fever, muscular rigidity, altered mental status, tachycardia, and autonomic dysfunction. It can then lead to change in mental status and consciousness, and can be a life-threatening emergency, treated only by discontinuing all neuroleptics and treating the symptoms supportively, sometimes with close monitoring in an intensive care unit.

Neuroleptic Malignant Syndrome (NMS)

A severe, although rare, side effect of neuroleptic treatment. It begins with rigidity or worsening in psychiatric symptoms despite increases in medication. Some of the warning signs are fast heart beat, high fluctuating blood pressure, tremors, sweating and fever. Cessation of neuroleptic therapy is the only treatment. It is a serious medical emergency that requires immediate attention.

Some medications such as benztropine and trihexyphenidyl (Artane®), which are an anticholinergic and an antihistaminic, respectively, are used solely for the

Metabolic syndrome

A collection of metabolic risk factors that includes elevated blood pressure, dyslipidemia, decreased glucose tolerance, and weight gain, especially in the abdomen. It sometimes develops as a side effect of medication use.

What Is the Metabolic Syndrome?

The **metabolic syndrome** is characterized by a group of metabolic risk factors that develops in one person. They include:

- Being overweight, and particularly the deposition of excessive fat tissue around the abdominal region
- Lipid disorders consisting of high blood triglycerides, low HDL cholesterol, and high LDL cholesterol, which in turn foster
  - Fatty deposits in arteries
  - Elevated blood pressure
- Insulin resistance or glucose intolerance
- A prothrombotic state of high fibrinogen or plasminogen activator inhibitor–1 in the blood
- A proinflammatory state with elevated C-reactive protein in the blood

People with the metabolic syndrome are at increased risk of coronary heart disease and stroke, peripheral vascular disease, and type 2 diabetes mellitus.

tremors and stiffness; but despite using these drugs, most patients on the older drugs still had visible effects. The main treatments for the metabolic syndrome are lowering cholesterol using statin drugs as well as controlling lipids in the diet, lowering blood pressure, and controlling diabetes and high blood sugar levels. Some trials of the oral antidiabetic medication, metformin, have shown usefulness for this side effect of some neuroleptics. For the drooling caused particularly by clozapine, sometimes glycopyrrolate (Robinul®), an anticholinergic agent, may be of help, although this too can have side effects.

35. How long does medication have to be taken?

Taking medication for schizophrenia is similar to taking medication for high blood pressure. Although someone who has only one episode of a psychosis should have a closely monitored trial without medications after being free of symptoms for one year, in 90% or more of these cases, the illness does reoccur within the first five years if medication is stopped. Thus, treatment is generally long-term and is considered necessary for the first decade after symptoms have appeared. If some symptoms, even residual negative ones, are still apparent, medication should be taken indefinitely. With recovery, the medication can be slowly tapered after several years and stopped. Not enough research is yet available to determine how long people need to take preventive medication long after the symptoms are gone and who will (or will not) benefit from a lifetime of medications.

36. Are long-acting injectables more helpful than oral medications?

Injectable long-acting neuroleptics (also called depot injectable medications) have long been used for chronic patients who are only maintainable in the community when they do not have to remember to take their daily doses of medication. These have included haloperidol decanoate and fluphenazine decanoate. Recently, there have been a few new, long-acting injectable medications made from the second-generation compounds that have been introduced on the clinical market. These include ones for risperidone (Risperdal Consta® given every 2 weeks) and its active metabolite paliperidone (Invega Sustenna® given every 4 weeks and just recently has been approved for every 3 months), as well as olanzapine (Zyprexa Relprevv® given every 4 weeks) and aripiprazole (Abilify Maintena® given every 4 weeks). The olanzapine long-acting injectable particularly needs to have the patient monitored closely for at least 30 minutes after it's administered to make sure side effects of dizziness and significant drop in blood pressure do not occur, and thus this medication has not been a popular injectable. This alternate route of receiving antipsychotic medication is an important advance, as one of the biggest problems in treating schizophrenia is a lack of compliance with oral medications. Many patients, if they take their prescribed medications at all when they leave the hospital, often do not take as much or as frequently as prescribed and ultimately relapse or, at very least, do not improve as much as they could. Trials of long-acting injectables compared with oral medications taken together appear to show a superior benefit for injectables, and they appear to have a significant effect on preventing rehospitalization. These should be offered to patients in clinical practice much more than is now done.

37. Is electroconvulsive therapy (ECT) a treatment for schizophrenia?

Electroconvulsive therapy (ECT) used for treatment in both schizophrenia and depression has received bad press over the years. Some hospitals do not allow it, and doctors' privileges to use it are separate from their regular medical licenses and hospital privileges. Certainly, if this is a recommended treatment, the qualifications for the person performing the ECT should be known. However, this procedure is actually quite safe with anticonvulsant medication given at the same time. Controversy exists, however, as to its efficacy for schizophrenia. Most studies do not show clear long-term results, and ECT certainly does not prevent the patient from having a recurrence even if the acute episode subsides. After ECT, maintenance antipsychotic medication will need to be given. Hallucinations that persist and plague a patient daily despite even clozapine trials deserve a trial of ECT. In fact, ECT is generally thought to be a treatment of choice in clozapine nonresponders and is a safe alternative to adding multiple other medications. One of the reasons to give ECT rather than antipsychotic medication as the first treatment of choice is to avoid the side effects of medication. This is less of an issue now with the advent of the newer medications that have relatively minimal side effects. One side effect of ECT is memory loss, and whether this loss is permanent is unclear. Nevertheless, ECT is more commonly given as the last resort in patients with schizophrenia when they have particularly comorbid depressive, manic, or violent symptoms that do not respond to usual medications.

Electroconvulsive therapy (ECT)

A type of treatment that gives a series of electrical shocks to regions of the brain given in sessions that are separated by several days. The only known side effect is memory loss subsequent to the treatment.

Max Fink (1999), a well-known authority on ECT, has written a helpful book about its uses. In it, he describes the beneficial effect of ECT for what he calls "the thought disorders"—the delusional/hallucinatory and language disorganization symptoms that occur predominantly in schizophrenia, but also in other illnesses as well. The number of ECT treatments, however, that is needed to alleviate these symptoms is larger than that for depression (as many as 15 to 25), and it may take longer for the ECT to reach its effect. In addition, if a course of ECT is not repeated, then relapse often occurs. A minimum of six months of treatment is recommended (Fink, 1999). The failure of ECT for schizophrenia that psychiatrists and families perceive could be due to a lack of continuation of the treatment rather than a lack of its usefulness.

A combination of ECT and antipsychotic medication may be more efficacious than either alone. Dr. Fink describes the mechanism as one in which the ECT can increase the ability for the medication to enter the neuronal cell membranes and thus exert its physiologic effect. The patient then might also require a smaller dose of the medication and be less likely to experience its side effects. Nevertheless, few psychiatrists use ECT today for schizophrenia, and they are generally not taught to do so in medical school. Only some residencies provide such training, as it is not a requirement for certification.

38. What is transcranial magnetic stimulation (TMS), and what can it do?

Transcranial magnetic stimulation (TMS) is a new treatment that has gained much popularity recently and has shown proven efficacy for suppressing active auditory hallucinations. TMS utilizes an electromagnet placed on the scalp that generates magnetic-field pulses roughly the strength of an MRI scan. The magnetic pulses stimulate a small area on the surface of the brain about the size of a quarter. Low-frequency (one pulse per second) TMS has been shown to induce small, sustained reductions in activity in the part of the brain that has been stimulated. Thus, studies have shown that if the part of the temporal lobes thought to be active in auditory hallucinations is stimulated, active hallucinations cease—at least temporarily. This is a novel treatment that is certainly worthwhile to try for treatment-resistant hallucinations, although currently not many physicians offer this as a treatment because they have not yet invested in the required equipment. More studies will also be needed to determine whether enough treatments over a period of time can permanently suppress the hallucinations or continued application will be needed. Finally, because it is so new, the side effects of this treatment are not yet clear.

39. What is cognitive behavioral therapy?

Cognitive behavioral therapy (CBT) has become a popular treatment for many emotional and behavioral traits. For schizophrenia, it has recently become a popular adjunct to medication at a time when the patient is stabilized but has a baseline of functional disturbances that are not alleviated by medication. In addition, some studies find it effective in delaying the onset of schizophrenia by treatment with CBT alone during the prodrome. Its use is now becoming more frequent and widespread for all stages in the schizophrenia spectrum.

CBT has two components: behavioral and cognitive. Behavior therapy is supposed to weaken the connections between troublesome situations and an individual's reactions to them. The reactions are such emotions as fear, depression, or rage and other self-defeating or self-damaging behavior. The cognitive aspect of the therapy focuses on changing thought patterns in order to change the emotional state and thus behavior. CBT has been used successfully in conditions such as depression, panic or anxiety disorders, and phobias and post-traumatic stress disorder. The basis for CBT in schizophrenia is that the disorder consists of a circumscribed set of irrational beliefs, and thus, easily learned techniques can alleviate the impact of those beliefs on one's daily life. The CBT therapists work to make patients aware that their thinking patterns are distorted and then train them to change these patterns by a process called "cognitive restructuring." This is different from psychodynamic psychotherapy, which instead tries to make patients understand why they behave the way they do and assumes that with understanding comes change. CBT does not involve understanding why one behaves a certain way, but uses behavior modification techniques to produce change in behavior. Some of these techniques include behavioral homework assignments that encourage patients to try new responses to difficult situations. Another is called "cognitive rehearsal," where a patient imagines a difficult situation and the therapist guides him or her through dealing with it. Patients may also keep a journal of their thoughts, feelings, and actions, although this may be difficult for patients with schizophrenia. The therapist also will use conditioning (positive reinforcement) and systematic desensitization from fears. Treatment is relatively short in comparison to some other forms of psychotherapy, usually lasting no longer than 16 weeks. Although many insurance plans provide reimbursement for cognitive behavioral therapy services, they may not yet reimburse for this treatment in schizophrenia.

Several organizations specialize in CBT in the United States and are listed in the Appendix. In the United Kingdom, Dr. Douglas Turkington at the University of Newcastle upon Tyne and Dr. Til Wykes at the Institute of Psychiatry in London, as well as others, have written books on this topic (e.g., Turkington & Turkington, 1995; Reeder and Wykes, 2005). More and more therapist are learning these techniques today, and thus almost every metropolitan area in the United States has someone available who is practicing CBT.

Beyond CBT, cognitive remediation, in general, can also be helpful for patients who have had comorbid traumatic brain injuries and post-traumatic stress disorder. Schizophrenia itself is now known to be associated with cognitive deficits. It particularly works on developing skills through specific drills for deficits in various areas of cognition, such as memory, being able to plan tasks, and learning new things. Thus, any kind of cognitive training program can be of great benefit for better functioning and thus quality of life.

40. Can a specific diet help, or using vitamin and fish oil supplements?

Unfortunately, throughout the years, there have been proponents of the idea that something in the diet (e.g., too much sugar, too much gluten, aspartame, or pesticides sprayed on field-grown food, as well as not enough **fish oils**) could cause schizophrenia. Popular "natural" or "alternative health" organizations stress that dietary

Fish oil

A common name for compounds derived from fish that contain omega-3 fatty acids.

changes would rid the body of toxins that cause schizophrenia, and they unfortunately encourage patients with schizophrenia to discontinue neuroleptic medications. In the past, more often than now, families would turn to these organizations often out of desperation, particularly when their relative was in a particularly severe state and control by medication was difficult. These organizations have been dangerous because they propose plans that have not been substantiated by rigorous research studies or treatment trials. You can still today find many websites and treatment centers that encourage these alternative treatments, although they are not as prevalent as they were a couple of decades ago.

Celebrities, who serve as role models, unfortunately are also prone to trying these unconventional treatments and publicize them (e.g., Margot Kidder, the movie star who acted in the Superman series). Margot had a severe, highly publicized psychotic episode several years ago that led her to become homeless for a while. She claims that medications were not the answer for her. She appeared on a well-known television talk show recounting how vitamin and mineral therapies have made her symptom-free and that Dr. Abram Hoffer, who introduced her to this regimen, saved her life. Dr. Hoffer, who passed away in 2009, was well known for his vitamin cocktails—which have never been substantiated with scientific treatment trials. Nevertheless, he maintained a faithful following for many years in Saskatchewan, Canada. His institute still exists and is now run by his followers as a vitamin information center (http://www.orthomolecularvitamincentre.com/about.php). Large doses of vitamin B3 (niacin) were the mainstay of his treatment. This is based on the knowledge that niacin is converted to nicotinamide adenine dinucleotide, an important coenzyme for facilitating various metabolic processes in the body. Niacin also has antihistaminic (antiallergenic) properties. Thus, Hoffer's assumption was that "brain allergies" are responsible to some degree for schizophrenia and its symptoms. Part of his regime was a reduced sugar and junk-food diet, which he said requires more niacin to metabolize (a claim that is also unsubstantiated). He also claimed that people with schizophrenia make a substance in their brain that serves as an endogenous hallucinogen and that niacin serves to reduce this toxin in the body, but again, there is *no evidence to support this*. To summarize, no scientific studies can substantiate any of Dr. Hoffer's claims, and in general, for people with schizophrenia, this treatment does more harm than good if it is thought of as an alternative for neuroleptic medications.

Another recognized pioneer in this field was David Horrobin, who has also since passed away. His area of research had been the clinical use of gamma-linolenic acid (GLA), an omega-3 derivative of an essential oil. It is present in the evening primrose, borage, and black currant seeds. He was one of the first to claim benefits from GLA in treating disease conditions of the nervous system. During his lifetime, he founded Scotia Pharmaceuticals and later Laxdale, Ltd. in Scotland and the journals *Medical Hypotheses* and *Prostaglandins, Leukotrienes, and Essential Fatty Acids.* While his journals are still active today, the 2 pharmaceutical companies are not: Scotia collapsed in 2001 and Laxdale was sold after his death in 2003 to the Amarin Corporation and is now known as Amarin Neuroscience Ltd. Dr. Horrobin was an energetic promoter of evening primrose oil in the treatment of schizophrenia and represented his company in campaigning vigorously for renowned senior scientists to conduct trials of its use. To date, some small studies suggest that it might be weakly beneficial as an adjunct to conventional medication in persons who do not completely respond to their normal treatment regime, but many studies have failed to find such an effect. His own controversial trials were under way at the time that he developed a malignant lymphoma, from which he died in 2003. He was an extremely engaging and convincing personality, who has had little following to explore his hypotheses further since his untimely death.

One other area where nutrition offers value for the schizophrenia patient is in consideration of vitamin D intake. Low vitamin D levels have been studied extensively and found to be present in a variety of neuropsychiatric illnesses as well as other medical conditions. This is certainly not surprising, given that vitamin D has a major effect on early brain development and growth. Low vitamin D levels during pregnancy and neonatally have been found in some studies to correlate to later development of schizophrenia. However, treatment with vitamin D has never been found in controlled trials to have a significant effect on schizophrenia symptoms. Nevertheless, examining vitamin D levels in patients with schizophrenia, particularly in winter months when less sunlight is available for absorbing vitamin D naturally, and then remedying low levels may have a positive effect in supplementing standard medication regimes, as vitamin D is known to modulate dopamine transmission and thus may possibly facilitate the effect of antipsychotic medications, inasmuch as they act on brain dopamine receptors.

Finally, since it is now recognized that there is clear communication between the gastrointestinal tract and the brain through hormonal and immunological mechanisms, there is renewed interest in the effect of gluten in the diet on causing brain changes that can put one at high risk for schizophrenia. The hypothesis is that gluten sensitivity and anti-gluten antibodies formed during an immune response may contribute to the disorder. Celiac disease is a well-known example of intestinal inflammation that is associated with an autoimmune process in which the presence of gluten stimulates autoantibodies in the gut. Some epidemiological studies show a higher percentage of celiac disease in people with schizophrenia. With renewed interest in the presence of inflammation at the onset of illness, this could be one association worth further focus. However, while there are anecdotal reports of removing gluten from the diets of people with schizophrenia leading to recovery, these claims currently are not substantiated by any large, carefully performed treatment trials.

41. Can individual, group, or family therapy help?

Many types of psychotherapy are available. The major reason for someone to consider psychotherapy is that he or she is unable to help himself or herself to make progress functioning satisfactorily with family and friends and in an occupation, and would like to improve his/her quality of life. People with schizophrenia benefit most from help with practical issues. Group therapy not only can be a helpful mechanism to improve one's condition but it can help the patient learn how to handle social interactions as well. The most useful type of therapy for patients with chronic schizophrenia supplements long-term neuroleptic medication and guides the patient to be able to manage the complexity of his or her daily activities. Learning how to reach attainable goals through positive reinforcement and encouragement is far more useful than insight-oriented psychodynamic therapy, which is more important for nonpsychotic individuals. Often this therapeutic setting can be provided best by psychiatric social workers.

Family therapy grew out of the many psychodynamic treatments that reached their peak in the 1970s. Two main principles were involved: The first is that there were communication disturbances within the family that led to confusion in the affected individual and which resulted in the symptoms of schizophrenia, and the second is that the patient is not the individual brought for treatment but rather the family unit as a whole. In general, the family therapy movement has caused a lot of damage to the well-being of families and to the relationship between the caregivers and consumers. Parents were told (or at least it was implied) that they were somehow at fault, and they did not want to be blamed. They needed help to deal with all the management issues that occur when a family member has a serious mental illness. Thus, this strained the relationship between families and the medical community, and it has taken many years to regain the trust that is needed for families to support the pharmacotherapy that is essential to treat those individuals with schizophrenia.

PART 3

Genetic Risk

"Mendel had painstakingly backcrossed pollen and egg cells from the common pea plant to reach a better understanding of inheritance. Mendel had recorded . . . his findings in a two-part lecture in 1865 . . . and then was all but ignored for the rest of his life . . . but rediscovered by Bateson in May 1900. Nearly a century after the debate over Mendelism that set the stage for contemporary genetics, almost every part of our modern understanding of how the world works—the relationship between parent and offspring . . . and the commonalities among all living things—can in a large measure be traced back to that startling spring of 1900, when anything was possible."

— Robin Marantz Henig (2000),
*The Monk in the Garden**

Is schizophrenia inherited?

Should I adopt a baby whose birth parent had schizophrenia?

If someone related to me has schizophrenia, what are my chances of getting it?

What are the chances of my children getting schizophrenia if my partner has a relative with it as well?

More . . .

42. Is schizophrenia inherited?

On April 14, 1930, four identical quadruplets weighing from 3 to 4 pounds 8 ounces were born by natural birth after a short labor and were placed in incubators. Although their childhood achievements varied, they grew up close with much societal attention until, within 6 months of each other in their early adulthood, they all had acute psychotic episodes that were eventually diagnosed as schizophrenia. Their notoriety as four genetically identical individuals who all had schizophrenia led to their being brought to the NIMH Laboratory of Psychology in the 1950s to be studied by a well-known group of investigators interested in searching for the causes of schizophrenia, and particularly in pursuing the genes versus environment or "nature versus nurture" controversy. Every test in use at that time, from the Rorschach to conventional electroencephalograms (EEGs), was given to the Genain Quadruplets, the name they were called to disguise their true identity. The investigators, David Rosenthal and Seymour Kety, first director of NIMH, went on from there to design adoption studies to be conducted in Denmark and produced pioneering data that turned the thinking of the time around from environmental to genetic/biological causes. There were also studies of twins at NIMH, such as those studied by the psychologist David Shakow, who developed many theories about environment and development of people who get schizophrenia. David Rosenthal, however, was the one that particularly developed a relationship with the family of the quadruplets, giving them the name "Genain," meaning "bad blood" and pseudonyms as Nora, Iris, Myrna, and Hester (representing NIMH) so that he could publish his findings but maintain the family's privacy. Again in 1979, after publication of the Kety-Rosenthal adoption studies and international recognition of the implications of these results, the Genains, then almost age 50, were brought back to NIMH to the laboratory of neuropsychopharmacology to be examined for abnormalities in all of the biological markers that were claimed to be important for schizophrenia at the time. I was privileged to be a young postdoctoral fellow in charge of managing the procedures and caring for these women during their two-month stay on the inpatient research ward. At that time, David Rosenthal accompanied them to NIMH, but quickly faded into the background, as he was dealing with his own newly diagnosed Alzheimer's disease.

During the period of getting to know these women, their fears, and variety of similar delusions and hallucinations, I also came to know the kind, silent face of Dr. Rosenthal, whose personal copy of his book was later taken off his office shelf and presented to me for my service to the Genains in his absence. Whether we learned anything biologically useful from working intensely with the Genains during that period was questionable, but the experience left a deep impression in my memory: No family could have such bad luck as to have all four of their children diagnosed with schizophrenia *unless the illness was genetic*. My later mentor in psychiatric genetics, Elliot S. Gershon, remarked during that time, when I commented on his lack of investment in our studies of the Genains, that I had gotten myself an "*N* of one," meaning essentially only one case study, nothing more, because these women all shared the identical DNA sequences, and that nothing fruitful could come out of such a genetic comparison study of any scientific rigor. Of course, he was ahead of the times and was correct, already a pioneer himself in more extensive psychiatric genetic research.

The thought that schizophrenia is inherited dates back to early 20th-century descriptions of the condition (*Dementia Praecox* by Emil Kraepelin). He estimated that "defective heredity," as he called it, was prominent and present in over 70% of cases (Kraepelin, 1907). From his early writings on, large family studies were conducted throughout Europe, particularly to estimate the amount of illness in close family members of individuals with schizophrenia. In general, they were consistent with the notion that there was an excess risk for schizophrenia to close relatives (siblings, offspring) of approximately 10%, but that the risks fell dramatically in more distant relatives, such as aunts, uncles, and cousins. The highest risks, however, were shown to be present in **monozygotic twin** pairs based on a series of independent twin studies. The biggest dilemma in psychiatric genetics today, however, is the attempt to explain why, although the risk to monozygotic twins is highest of any recorded risk factor for schizophrenia, it falls considerably short of 100% (i.e., only 50% on average). One-hundred percent similarity is what would be expected if two individuals share an identical genetic makeup. Although most people seem to think that the low 50% concordance rate among identical twins is evidence for environmental interactions with genes, modification of gene expression by internally controlled molecular mechanisms has not been excluded.

Monozygotic twins

Twins born at the same time who originate from the splitting of the same egg after it has been fertilized. The DNA is identical in both twins; and thus the twins are sometimes referred to as identical.

The turning point in schizophrenia research, and probably the most important data collection and results of the 20th century in this field, came from the carefully planned and executed adoption studies of Seymour Kety and David Rosenthal using Danish case registries to identify parents with schizophrenia and their offspring (Rosenthal and colleagues, 1968) and adopted-at-birth children who developed schizophrenia, comparing diagnoses in their biological and adoptive relatives (Kety and colleagues, 1968). As a group, regardless of the study design, these investigators showed that an excess of schizophrenia was present in the biological relatives of individuals with schizophrenia, but not the adoptive relatives. These data were fuel for the nature/nurture debates of the time and initiated great changes in the focus of research on schizophrenia from the 1970s to the present. They turned the corner from support for "nurture" to support for primarily "nature." Initially, when these results were reported, the leadership of academic psychiatry departments throughout the United States was predominantly made up of psychoanalysts, and this was true of the most prestigious of training institutes. Soon these individuals, however, were replaced by biologically-oriented chairpersons who led a new era of research—and the field of biological psychiatry was born.

43. Should I adopt a baby whose birth parent had schizophrenia?

There is about a 10-fold increase in risk over the general population for a child to develop schizophrenia when a parent has been affected. Thus, adoption of such a child should be treated with caution. The child may appear normal for many years, but then tragically become ill after many years of devotion from adoptive parents. The decision is personal but should be considered seriously, at least until medications become available that can be administered early on to prevent a full-blown illness. Adoption agencies should at least now inform prospective families of this history and, if not, the prospective parents should request the information. We now know much more about the genetics of diseases that were previously not recognized as inherited or biological. It may be useful to take this information either to a research psychiatrist who knows genetics for consultation or a genetic counselor who is trained in these issues. While it is highly unlikely that genetic testing will be useful for schizophrenia, other diseases at least may be ruled out by genetic testing and thus before adoption, testing could be warranted.

44. If someone related to me has schizophrenia, what are my chances of getting it? What are the chances of my children getting schizophrenia if my partner has a relative with it as well?

Children would share the same amount of genetic material with a parent's uncle as with their own first cousin (parent's sibling's child), and the risk for schizophrenia in both cases would be very small (**Table 1**) and almost the same as in the general population. However, if the relative is a closer one, such as a parent, sister or brother, chances are much higher, and in a broad sense of who is affected with illness, it can be as high as 10%.

If the illness is present in both sides of the family, then the chances of a child becoming affected would be greater, although there are no clear statistics to say how much greater. In addition, these are only general risk statistics, and thus what happens in each individual family will vary. We do not know what the real risks are until the actual genes that lead to a predisposition for schizophrenia are identified and their mechanisms for producing disease determined. The risks shown in Table 1 are based only on prevalence rates from the older, large family studies that exist. Moreover, one has to consider that since the 1980s, there have been newer, carefully controlled family studies using the American Psychiatric Association DSM diagnostic categories. In these studies, the risk to any close family relative is still elevated, but is considerably lower than in previous reports (on average, about 7 to 8%), and again, they do not tell us what may happen in the individual family.

45. If I have an identical twin with schizophrenia, but I am well, what are my children's chances of having schizophrenia?

According to some twin studies, it appears that the risk for schizophrenia to offspring of well versus ill identical twins is the same and would be similar to the risk

Table 1 Familial Risks for Schizophrenia in Relatives of People with Schizophrenia.

Relationship	% Chance of Developing Schizophrenia	% Chance of Developing an Illness with a Dominant Inheritance
Identical twins	48	100
Nonidentical twins	17	50
Siblings	9	50
Children	13	50
Parents	6	50
Grandchildren	5	25
Nieces and nephews	4	25
Aunts and uncles	2	25
First cousins	2	12.5
Unrelated individuals	1	N/A*

* Dependent on the prevalence of the risk gene in the population.

Modified from Gottesman II [1991].

to children of an affected person in general (i.e., 13%; Table 1). These studies, however, have been flawed in design and limited in their numbers. People with schizophrenia, particularly men, have fewer offspring than those who do not have schizophrenia; thus, the number of offspring of ill versus well identical twins will not likely be the same. Because of the difficulties in obtaining and studying identical twins where one has schizophrenia, the numbers for comparisons in these studies are small. This issue is thus still controversial but is an important one. If these rates were equal, then one assumes that something in the genetic sequence (identical DNA sequence) must be what is crucial for schizophrenia susceptibility. If these rates really are unequal, although still in excess in the offspring of the co-twin without schizophrenia, then some modification of the defective gene's expression, either endogenously or by the environment, is likely to be taking place as well. Alternatively, there appear to be new clues from the use of the latest gene sequencing technology to date that have shown in at least one study of identical twins discordant for schizophrenia that genetic mutations in some parts of the body may be occurring after the twin embryos have split in the womb. Thus it is possible that a mutation in a crucial gene or genes is responsible for one of the twins developing schizophrenia. We hope that molecular genetic studies of twins will yield more definitive answers about this in the near future.

46. What chromosomal risk factors can increase one's risk for schizophrenia?

There are certain chromosomal anomalies that have been found to be associated with a high incidence of schizophrenia, as well as other psychiatric illnesses. Particularly, having an extra X **chromosome** (Klinefelter's syndrome in males and Triple X syndrome in females) appears to have an association with schizophrenia. However, while the risk is greater than that to people with normal chromosomal karyotypes, it is still very small.

Chromosome
A structure present in the nucleus of every cell of the body of any living thing containing genes. It is shaped like a long cylinder separated into two arms that are held together in the approximate middle by a structure called the centromere. The two arms have been named "p" and "q" arms.

Another anomaly is a large deletion that appears on chromosome 22 and is known as the Velo-Cardio-Facial Syndrome (VCFS). As indicated, these individuals have characteristic pathology that has nothing to do with the brain, but as many as 50% of them are also diagnosed with schizophrenia.

47. What are the methods used to find gene defects that are associated with schizophrenia?

Before the late 1980s, the biological research that was pursued on the genetics of schizophrenia was largely conducted by examining factors in blood, urine, and cerebral spinal fluid that were different in chronic patients with schizophrenia compared with controls. These numerous studies produced nothing consistent, and in fact many of those early positive findings were eventually found to be due to either the medications the patients were taking, their dietary differences, or the effects of institutionalization. When the field of molecular genetics began to explode in the early 1980s by identifying multiple, highly variable markers spread throughout the genome for specific genes, it became clear that these markers could be used to map the chromosomal location of different diseases. By identifying genes in the specific mapped location, researchers could then find a variation in a gene that leads to that specific disease. These methods then began to be applied to psychiatric disorders with genetic susceptibility, particularly schizophrenia.

Many research groups worldwide began to evaluate families that, by virtue of having more than one sibling with schizophrenia, were considered ideal for these chromosomal **linkage** studies. The principles of genetic linkage studies are as follows: Our genes are organized in predetermined locations on pairs of 23 chromosomes (46 total). One of each pair is inherited from each parent. During reproduction, however, an independent assortment of the maternal and paternal genes on chromosome pairs exists so that the farther away genes are from each other on each chromosome, the more the likelihood that different combinations of genes are inherited on the final chromosomes of the offspring of a mother–father pair. This is why no two siblings look alike unless they are identical twins and come from the same egg and sperm during fertilization. If there are known, highly variable markers that could be spaced out and attached to the string of sequences of DNA from genes and the spaces surrounding them, across all chromosomes, one could then see which variations in DNA are present in each individual and trace the inheritance of variations found with these markers down generations in families (**Figure 1**).

Linkage

A genetic term that signifies a relationship between two or more genes on the same chromosome that are relatively close together so that sometimes the variations in the traits each represent are inherited together in the same individual.

In each family, different variations in the markers for sequences will be present (because the mother has two and the father has two different ones), but it is the position of the sequences that the markers attach to on chromosomes that is important, not the exact variation in the marker. Think of maps of towns: We have street names that vary and are different. The unique names help us locate houses on the streets. We can find the house because it is located between two named street signs. So it is with a disease gene. It is not the marker itself that will cause an illness, but it is the gene for an illness that is close to a specific marker that is important. If an illness gene is close to that marker, it will tend to be transmitted with the marker down generations, and we then say it is "linked." It is said to be "mapped" near that marker. Thus, the people with illness within a family will all be likely to inherit that particular variation that the marker represents.

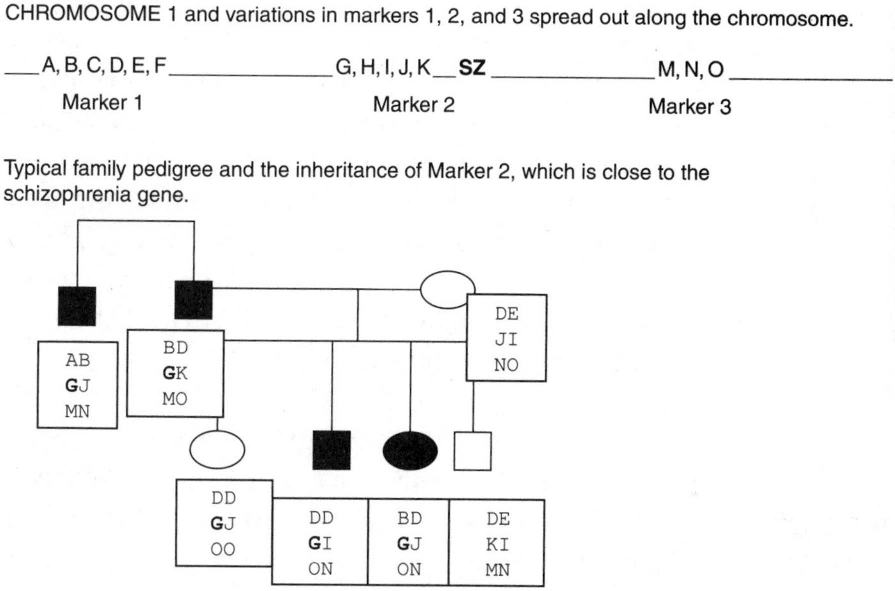

Figure 1 Illustration of linkage of schizophrenia to a chromosome if Marker 2 on chromosome 1 is linked to schizophrenia (SZ). Alleles (variations) for Marker 1 are A, B, C, D, E, F; alleles for Marker 2 are G, H, I, J, K; alleles for Marker 3 are M, N, O. The inheritance of a specific allele for each marker is represented under each individual in a box. Note that each individual inherits two alleles for each Marker (one from his/her mother and one from his/her father). Also note that all blackened individuals have schizophrenia and they have all inherited the same allele for Marker 2 because it is so close to the schizophrenia gene that whatever variant a person inherited for Marker 2 is inherited with the schizophrenia gene. In this family, the G allele appears to be inherited with schizophrenia.

Geneticists

Scientists who study the inheritance of traits in humans, animals or plants.

Geneticists, based on this information in families with multiple ill and well members, are capable of calculating how likely it is that a gene for illness is linked to a marker, given the pattern of marker inheritance that is observed in families such as the one illustrated in Figure 1. This method has been highly successful in the search to find genes for disorders known to be genetic, such as Huntington's chorea or phenylketonuria. A gene, such as one for schizophrenia, which may be only one of many that causes the same illness, and which may have a nontraditional, more complex mode of inheritance, is not so easy to find by this method. In fact, the irony is that over the past decade, there have been reports of many positive linkage findings for schizophrenia spread throughout all 23 chromosomes, and it has been difficult for researchers to tell which of these positives are true findings and which are falsely positive, having been only chance findings. The key to this dilemma will be to find strong gene candidates whose involvement makes sense given their known functions and to confirm these findings by other sources of evidence.

Microarray

This is an orderly arrangement of DNA samples to identify many genes at one time. They can contain thousands of genes on one small plate or "chip." An experiment with a single DNA chip or microarray can provide researchers information on thousands of genes simultaneously.

The explosion of new technology in molecular genetics in recent years has resulted in the development of RNA **microarrays** and gene chip microarrays. These have led to the ability to provide data using a very large number of markers (in the millions) and a large number of individual samples for a relatively small cost. In schizophrenia research over the last decade, there has been a remarkable trend for researchers to organize into large international consortiums to combine the samples collected into one huge collection that would enable the uncovering of common genetic variation present in the normal population that could put people at high risk for schizophrenia. The analyses from such a set of samples is called a "GWAS" or Genome-Wide Association

Study. The large consortium that has formed world-wide is called the Psychiatric Genomic Consortium (PGC) and is made up of several hundred schizophrenia investigators from all over the world. Together the PGC has more than 100,000 DNA samples at this writing. The latest results from such a GWAS recently published implicated over 108 genes that have variants elevating one's risk for schizophrenia—albeit a risk that is still small, at about 2% each. Investigators are now combining them into a so called "polygenic risk score" that quantifies one's risk for schizophrenia based on the number of these variants one actually inherits. Much more research is needed, however, to be able to use such a score in the clinic, and it is unlikely that the one currently being examined will be put to such use, since it is likely to pick up too many false positives; that is, it appears to detect risk correctly in only a small percentage of cases (some reports indicate as low as 3%). As of this writing, researchers are now collaborating to completely sequence the genome of large groups of people with schizophrenia comparing the sequence to controls. However, the amount of information produced is enormous, and how to interpret it all becomes very complex and may take a very long time.

Of all the genetic material in the human genome, only a very small amount of the DNA sequence actually leads to the production of proteins that, in turn, have a function in the body. The DNA that will be expressed is transferred into complementary sequences of messenger RNA (mRNA) that produce proteins critical to directing all bodily functions. This process is called gene expression. The process is complicated by many control mechanisms that enable the crucial timing of expression of genes and their turning on and off at different times in the lifespan of individuals. Gene expression throughout the genome can be examined on microarrays in a direct and comprehensive way, as can gene structural variation among individuals. Gene methylation (modification by methyl groups) that is responsible for turning on and off of gene expression can also be determined.

Microarray technology enables researchers to examine thousands of genes at once in the laboratory. The microarrays themselves are small slide or plate-like laboratory structures that support thousands of genes at fixed immobilized locations. The researcher places the gene markers in these locations in an orderly fashion, and thus, it is called an "array." If the expression of a gene is to be examined, the experiment is called "microarray expression analysis." If a gene is overexpressed in a certain disease state, then more of a sample of a sequence of expressed DNA will be present compared with control DNA. Arrays use fluorescent colors to quantify the amount of expression, and so if a particular gene expression is involved, it may be seen by expression of a different color. Similarly, the colors are different if structure is examined for different DNA bases or whether or not a segment is methylated.

In schizophrenia research, microarray expression studies have been carried out on postmortem brains of patients who had chronic schizophrenia. Many results have come out of these studies, but it is still too early to tell whether the findings are consistent and relate to the findings from the gene association and linkage studies. Some early expression studies implicate genes for neuronal connectivity and growth. These studies, however, have so far not been able to clarify the effects that medication intake and other problems of illness chronicity and aging have on differential gene expression. In addition, examining brains of older people after death may not be useful for finding genes that are only expressed during prenatal brain development and in childhood. Lastly, the large numbers of the PGC cannot be replicated in postmortem brain studies, the latter having very small numbers of samples by comparison.

48. What genes are currently implicated as risks for schizophrenia?

Before the recent GWAS studies, there were claims from several linkage studies that genes within linked regions that are known to be brain-expressed could be involved in susceptibility for schizophrenia. The exact nature of their roles has not been elucidated, although some have general relevance, particularly to glutamatergic neurochemical brain pathways that appear widespread throughout the brain, some of which have been thought to be relevant to schizophrenia. Others clearly are involved in brain growth during development.

In addition to the linkage and microarray studies, there are the so-called early candidate gene-association studies, where a specific variant in a gene is more frequent in populations of schizophrenic patients than in control populations. Many positive results have also come out of these studies because the standards for what constitutes a positive finding have not yet been agreed on by researchers in the field. What is interesting is that these were relatively small studies with many positive results. The recent GWAS are very large studies, yet they do not find many of these same candidate genes, but rather different ones. It may just be that the early findings were false positives, and thus the specific genes found earlier to be involved will not be named here.

The gene variants that appear to lead to greater risk for schizophrenia that resulted from the latest GWAS studies (Schizophrenia Working Group of the Psychiatric Genomics Consortium, 2014) are common variations in genes that do not lead to illness in most people. It is estimated that each individual genetic change that has been found to be associated with schizophrenia only confers a very small elevation in the risk (about 2%).

No pathological defect has been found in any of these genes—that is, a mutation has not been found in these genes that is present in people with schizophrenia and not in controls. There are a couple of exceptions to this. One comes from another kind of study that will be covered in Question 51—that is, there are also rare copy number variations (CNVs) in the DNA of some people that may in some rare families be major risk factors for illness. For the most part, however, these studies have not shown that within multiple families all those with schizophrenia have the putative rare variant, whereas those who do not have schizophrenia do not have it. Another exception comes from the sequencing of the genome in some large families with multiple ill members. In these families, mutations in a gene unique to each family seem to be present in all ill members and not the well ones. These mutations may be particularly interesting to pharmaceutical companies as a target for new drugs that can not only help that individual family but hopefully many others with the illness in general.

The list of putative common variants that are candidates for increasing the risk for schizophrenia, are in genes for brain growth factors, genes related to the growth and activity of the neurosynapse for neurochemical transmission in the brain, genes for neuroinflammation and the immune response in general, dopamine receptor genes, the physiological calcium-channel genes, multiple genes involved specifically in **glutamate** neurotransmission, and those involved with the nicotinic cholinergic receptor. At the time of this writing, many, if not all, of these claimed gene findings could be false-positive research findings, although patterns are clearly emerging with some replications as well. Definitive replication studies are urgently needed, although given the large numbers of samples already compiled worldwide as part of the PGC, these will not come easily.

Glutamate

An amino acid that is a building block of proteins. It is also by itself a major neurotransmitter in the brain (i.e., transmits information from cell to cell); by stimulating the activity of the cells, it excites them into activity.

49. Are any risk genes specific to schizophrenia, or are they implicated in other diseases as well?

Many of the genetic changes being associated with schizophrenia overlap with those of other diseases, such as autism, bipolar disorder, depression, and others. It may be that there will never be found that one particular genetic constellation is specific to schizophrenia, but rather that the genetic findings may ultimately generate a new classification of syndromes of psychiatric disorders, and the illness we call schizophrenia, as such, will be obsolete. That is one possibility that remains. Nevertheless, we are reminded that we can still clinically define a syndrome we call schizophrenia that has meaning for the questions outlined in this book, and is certainly an entity from which much suffering occurs.

50. How is it assumed that genes cause schizophrenia?

Neuronal transmission is maintained by complex interaction of several neurochemicals with specific receptors on nerve cells: Dopamine, serotonin, GABA, norepinephrine, glutamate, and acetylcholine. One possiblity is that some genes that control the balance of different neurotransmitters, ultimately cause schizophrenia by changing this balance; thus, their receptors have become targets for the development of pharmacotherapies, i.e., new drugs, many of which have mixed profiles for how they affect multiple types of receptors. However, just because a drug that blocks a specific receptor may suppress the illness, this does not suggest that an abnormality of the receptor is necessarily *responsible* for the illness. However, since most of the effective treatments for schizophrenia involve blocking dopamine D-2 receptors, it is not so surprising that the gene for the dopamine D-2 receptor was found to be one that was associated with increased risk for schizophrenia in the latest GWAS (see Question 47).

Another trend that has been noticed about the putative risk genes is some of them particularly converge on the neurochemical pathways for the neurotransmitter glutamate. Others, however, appear to have functions involved in developing neuronal structural networks, such as in aiding the migration of neurons during growth of the brain. Still others appear to be involved in the brain inflammatory response.

One possible scenario is that one or more genes are defective in a certain way and that these genes are turned on and off during different stages of the lifespan of an individual, perhaps even in an abnormal timing mechanism as well. Thus, during prenatal development, some brain structures may develop abnormally in a subtle way; during adolescence, neuronal connections may abnormally form, and during aging, neurons may age in an accelerated or abnormal way and inflammatory responses may be more crucial in response to the environment. In general, there will be less brain plasticity (**Figure 2**). All this is caused by abnormalities in likely several genes and/or their expression at different times during life and of different kinds during the lifespan.

Current research still has a long way to go in order to understand the lifetime trajectory of how and when gene expression contributes to schizophrenia. However, currently the tide is turning from focus on single genes to pathways and systems involving multiple genes. From there the field will then likely be able to turn to understanding the longitudinal dynamics of gene expression both in normal and abnormal functioning.

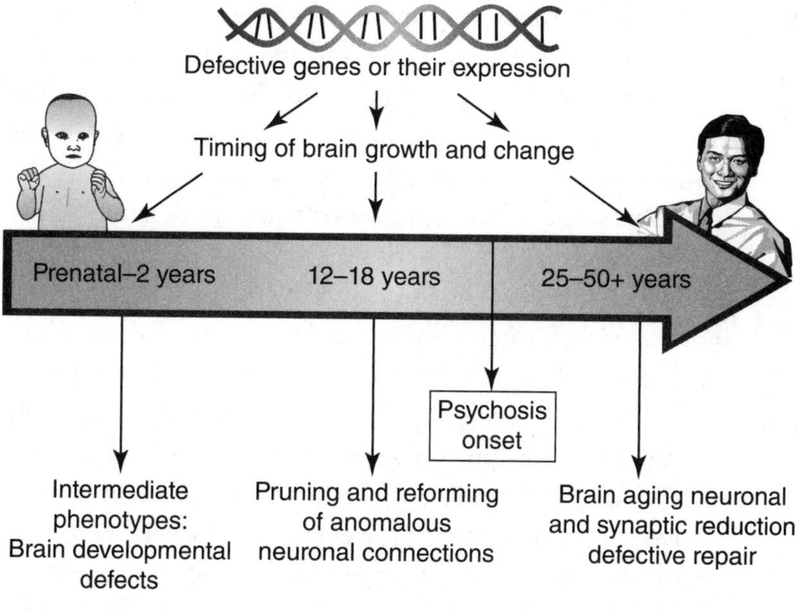

Figure 2 The concept that schizophrenia is a lifetime disorder with different genetically controlled events occurring at each stage by activation and deactivation of the same defective genes.

51. What do DNA copy number variations (CNVs) have to do with schizophrenia?

One theory is that the genetic mechanism for schizophrenia in part could be due to multiple rare mutations throughout the genome in genes relevant to brain growth and development or functioning in some way. These can either be inherited from parent to offspring or arise from a so-called mutational hotspot in the genome and spontaneously occur in the germline for one individual.

Human genome

The complete catalogue of genes and genetic variation in human DNA.

Copy number variations (CNVs)

Microduplications or microdeletion within genes that alter gene function.

This theory has been born out recently with the discovery that there are numerous segments that are duplicated throughout the genome. Segmental duplications are sections of DNA with near-identical sequence in the **human genome** (see **Figure 3**). Between these segments are genes. When maternal and paternal chromosomes come together during meiosis to form an embryo, the segments disrupt the proper pairing of chromosomes and either regions of genes are duplicated along the chromosome of the embryo or they are deleted. These microduplications or deletions have been dubbed **copy number variations** or **CNVs**, and the gene or genes within them may be malfunctioning as a result or disrupted. A significant increase in the general number of CNVs has been reported in the genome of people with schizophrenia in some recent large studies and some specific regions of the genome where they exist have been implicated. However, these observations are still in their infancy. It is not known what the pattern of CNVs are like within families, and this needs to be studied.

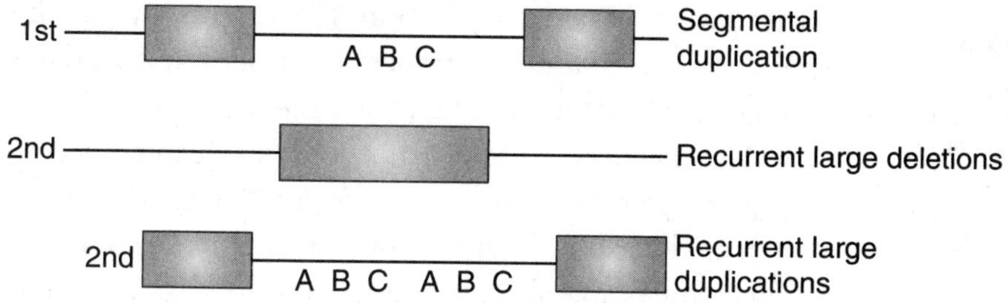

Figure 3 Segmental duplications and copy number variations. The line represents one chromosome, ABC = 3 different genes or portions of genes along the chromosome. 1st = 1st generation; 2nd = what may occur in offspring as a result of the segmental duplication. Either the region in between with genes A, B, and C is deleted or it is duplicated after recombination of maternal and paternal chromosomes to form the embryo.

52. What is an endophenotype for schizophrenia?

A **phenotype** is a trait or cluster of traits expressed by a gene, but not all phenotypes occur directly from gene activation and may actually be far down the path from what is directly produced by the gene. It is now thought that genes that cause schizophrenia likely act by affecting an "intermediate step" (or intermediate phenotype)—that is, directly causing a change in the brain that will then lead to a vulnerability for developing schizophrenia—but that the genetic defects themselves will not be directly responsible for the illness as a whole (**Figure 4**). The rules for what is an **intermediate phenotype** are that (1) the trait has to have been shown consistently to be abnormal in people who have schizophrenia compared with those that do not; (2) the trait must have been demonstrated to be inherited (i.e., run in families); (3) within families who have inherited the trait, it should be present in all individuals

Phenotype

The trait that is expressed by a gene. For example, having blue eyes or brown eyes would be phenotypes.

Intermediate phenotype

The trait in genetic terms that a gene is responsible for producing. For example, an intermediate phenotype for schizophrenia may be a change in the structure of the brain that in turn may put someone at risk to get schizophrenia. Also called **endophenotype**.

Endophenotype

A trait in genetic terms that a gene is responsible for producing and makes a person more vulnerable to getting an illness. Also called **intermediate phenotype** because it is intermediate between the gene and the clinical symptoms.

who have schizophrenia; (4) and lastly, it may also be present in well family members because despite having the genes for schizophrenia, the illness does not always develop. The term "endophenotype" has been coined to represent some trait formed within a person that is an "intermediate phenotype". Thus far, many brain structural changes and also changes in cognitive functioning, such as certain types of memory loss, have been candidates for **endophenotypes**, but at this time no one factor is clearly known to be intermediate between genes and the clinical manifestation of illness.

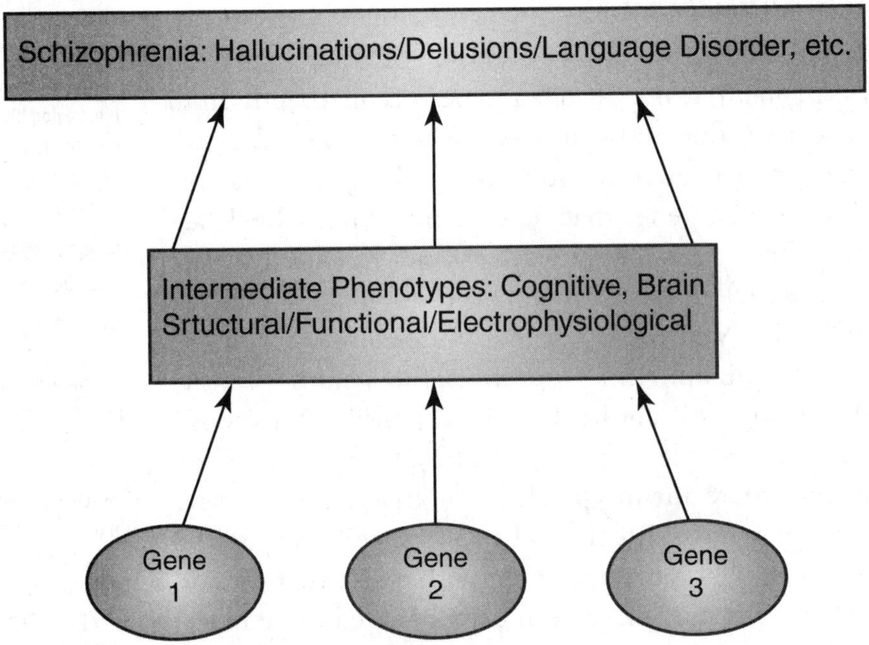

Figure 4 This diagram depicts how genes directly affect "intermediate phenotypes" that are a long the pathway toward influencing the development of schizophrenia.

53. *Are there lab tests to identify genetic risk for schizophrenia?*

It is possible to examine one's chromosomes in the laboratory (by performing what is called a high-resolution karyotype) and thus in the rare case of triple X (XXX) or Klinefelter's (XXY), these can be found. Usually a doctor will order these tests if there are other characteristics that may be abnormal in patients, such as lack of secondary sex characteristics. Certainly some CNVs that have been implicated in a few studies can be seen in the laboratory as well. However, just because it is possible, does not mean it should be done or that the results will be useful. Doctors may order many genetic tests from a reputable laboratory, but they are not helpful for diagnosis of future or current schizophrenia. In order to be a predictor for risk of illness, the laboratory test would have to have a high sensitivity (pick up most cases and not have too many false positives) and also have a high specificity for the illness. No laboratory test does this for schizophrenia.

54. *Should I order commercially available DNA tests for schizophrenia?*

You may not need to have a physician as the intermediary for obtaining such a "laboratory" test as you do with other conditions. Direct-to-consumer DNA testing has become quite popular and is readily available for a great number of genetic conditions by commercial companies one can find by simply searching the Internet. DNA can be obtained from from saliva or a blood sample, and this can be sent directly to the company as directed. You can also, of course ask your doctor to do so, but the same question needs to be answered—should you do this? Although you can find out whether or not you have inherited a high risk for a variety of neurological and medical conditions, at the time of this writing, schizophrenia is not one of them (see Question 53). If a commercial company does advertise "tests" for schizophrenia and other serious mental illnesses, such as bipolar disorder, one should be aware of the danger to misinterpretation of the results of these tests and not be tempted to order one. They are not reliable indicators of who will develop schizophrenia and may only cause harm to people's lives if any life decisions are based on what these tests show. These tests have little value, and there is no basis for their sale at this time, nor is there likely to be in the future. They are the "snake oil" of the new genetic era we find ourselves in after having had the human genome completely sequenced in laboratories.

The public should be wary of any commercial entity that advertises a test of any kind, genetic or otherwise, for schizophrenia. It is highly unlikely that a specific genetic defect will be helpful for testing people to see whether they have inherited the tendency for schizophrenia. This is because, given the highly nonspecific biological and clinical findings in schizophrenia, and knowing that having high-risk variants of specific genes only confers a small general risk for illness, no test of any one genetic variant will be likely to have enough sensitivity and specificity to be useful on a population basis for accurate testing. Even the Polygenic Risk Factor, which is calculated by adding together a lot of small risk gene variants, still does not account for a great enough risk to be a useful test in the laboratory. There will just be too many false positives and false negatives. It would be difficult to know what to do with the results, as most people having a positive test may never develop the disorder—and furthermore, if one had a negative finding, it would not mean that the disorder *wouldn't* develop, as there are several other genetic defects and causes that the test may not identify.

Regardless, any reported "test" will need to be thoroughly investigated in large trials before being used by the public or commercially. All signs so far indicate that the combination of individual risk genes is not going to lead to any application to clinical work that focuses on prediction of illness anytime soon. After genes are established that contribute to vulnerability, it is likely that their use will be confined to clarifying the scientific understanding of the mechanism for schizophrenia, which can then lead ultimately to the development of new medications.

55. Can DNA testing enable physicians to determine which medications to administer?

This could be a better eventual use of DNA sequence variation among individuals. Although variation in specific gene DNA may not be associated with the illness itself, the medications that suppress its symptoms may be responded to in different ways depending on the genetic makeup of each individual. For example, if some people have **enzymes** that have higher activity for inactivating a certain medication, then these people may need higher doses to get a clinical response than people with lower enzyme activity will need, or these simply may not be responders to that particular medication. Similarly, if other individuals have low activity of an inactivating enzyme, they may have the drug in their system longer and thus be more prone to side effects. It also may be possible in the future to predict whether

Enzymes
Proteins in the body that digest other substances through biochemical reactions. They are the "tools" of metabolism.

someone will respond to a drug such as clozapine by what alleles they carry for a specific gene. These genetic tests may also be important to predict when someone will not respond to certain medications, so that the medication they are likely to respond to can be given earlier in the course of their illness. For example, if we could predict who will not respond to conventional neuroleptics but would respond to clozapine, it would then be possible to give clozapine earlier in the course of illness and prevent severe chronic continuation of symptoms. These factors, once established, could be available to clinicians so that they can tailor treatment with the many available drugs to each individual's unique genetic makeup. These principles belong to the new burgeoning field of "pharmacogenetics" (now also called "precision medicine") and hold promise for the future but will need several years of development to be useful.

56. How can genetic research provide new treatments?

As stated previously here, an understanding of the biology of schizophrenia can only lead to better treatments, ones that can be given earlier, before pronounced clinical symptoms appear. Drug companies need what they call "targets" for drugs to act on and change, whether it is a neurochemical receptor blockade, growth of cells, activation of brain regions on an MRI scan, or a change in an EEG pattern. In turn, a change in the targets need to be shown to be associated with improvement with a new drug. Consumers, however, need to be aware that developing drugs to targets takes a long time and is a complicated process. It takes many years for pharmaceutical companies to develop and test new drugs, and for every compound that the companies explore, many are abandoned for various reasons before they ever reach the market.

57. What are the ethical concerns about genetic testing? Do those with genes for schizophrenia face discrimination?

The ideas of "genes," "genetics," and specific patterns of inheritance grew out of the discoveries of the late 1800s and early 1900s, and thus the field of "genetics" was born, gradually evolving into what we know of its science today. With it, however, also grew the notion of "eugenics" (i.e., that if genetic defects caused undesirable traits, one could eliminate these traits in society). Sterilization became an acceptable procedure for people who were considered "genetic undesirables" in society, which included those with mental retardation and also psychiatric disturbances. Although little is publicized about these times, the Cold Spring Harbor Laboratories (Long Island, New York), today a center of excellence in molecular genetics, was then a "hotbed" in the United States for the eugenics movement.

The Holocaust of the mid-twentieth century looms high on the list of human atrocities inflicted on our fellow man in recent times. It was characterized by a program for the extermination of people for the sole reason that their heritage included Jewish ancestry, as well as others considered "undesirable" because of their genetic make-up. For this reason, there was considerable participation of German psychiatrists at that time in the extermination of psychotic patients in psychiatric hospitals. In Germany alone, at least five such hospitals were equipped with gas chambers and connected incinerators during the years from 1938 to 1940. Preservation of the building for such procedures can be seen today in the Hadamar Psychiatric Hospital, a short distance from Frankfurt, where a museum depicts the scene of busloads of patients being delivered each day down to the "showers" by one door and then out the opposite door as corpses to the autopsy table for the academic neuropathologist/psychiatrist to have an opportunity to examine the postmortem brain before incineration. Eventually—but not before 10,000 patients were exterminated in this way at Hadamar—the Bishop of Muenster spoke out about this suspected atrocity, and Hitler was forced to abandon this practice in the psychiatric hospitals. Nevertheless, the doctors and nurses in these hospitals continued various methods of euthanasia by injection and starvation until the end of World War II and the fall of the Nazi party. This is a striking example of the extreme misuse of genetic information. One may simply read this and say that it cannot happen again and that perhaps the lesson from history has been learned. But has it?

We are part of a different scientific age now. The explosion of new technology in the field of genetics has enabled us to have available methods of identifying variations in almost all genes in the human genome. What will be done with this information now that we have it needs continual discussion about its ethical implications and legislation.

The science fiction movie *Gattaca* (1997) is an illustration about what could go wrong. The movie hypothesizes a future with two classes of human beings: Those whose genes were "enhanced" in utero (i.e., deleterious variants were replaced with "better" ones) and those individuals who were born of natural unions between men and women. The latter are discriminated against, cannot get professional jobs, and are forbidden to marry those who were enhanced. Everyone carries his or her own DNA card, which is proof of one's identity, and it may be used to their advantage or disadvantage. Could this happen in reality?

Scientifically, no barriers to such a future exist. Already, in vitro fertilization offers the opportunity to allow parents to choose the sex of a baby; "gene editing" offers the possibility of changing other characteristics, perhaps without limit. What we do with new genetic information must be open for serious discussion.

Scientists must always take social responsibility for their new discoveries. Some families are happy to know that schizophrenia has a strong genetic component because then they know that it has been out of their control and that their behavior was not responsible for making someone ill in their family. Other families, in contrast, see that they have somehow been stigmatized and are passing on "bad genes." There is also the concern that people will want genetic testing before mating so as not to raise a child who is likely to get this illness or will think twice about marrying someone with a family history of this illness, despite scientific knowledge that the excess genetic risk is low and not understood. In addition, once a test result is available, despite privacy laws, if they appear in a medical record, other people may be able to obtain the information and this has implications for whether health insurance companies may provide coverage, and potential employers may hire a person or promote that person to a role of leadership and responsibility. You could envision numerous such scenarios coming from superficial knowledge that schizophrenia is genetic. Scientists in collaboration with lawmakers must develop legislation that prevents the misuses of genetic data to label individuals.

Psychiatrists in the eugenic movement of the mid 1900s used superficial genetic statistics to suggest that sterilizing and then exterminating people who had "inherited" mental illness would be best for society. Thus, we need to learn from history and proceed cautiously given the historical potential for use of genetic information to scapegoat religious and other groups. Many other possibilities of abuse of genetic information are looming in the future, since with advanced technology, we can now determine the variants of genes that are present in embryos. What harm will we be doing in the future if certain variants are not allowed to continue according to the rules of evolution and natural selection?

In summary, the movie *Gattaca* was provocative and went relatively unnoticed. It was a startling look at what could happen in the future. The "genetically enhanced" population of people in the movie may be more of a reality, given today's technology, than simply science fiction. Other abuses have to do with the public use of genetic information if it is known at birth. Could insurance companies and life insurance salespersons refuse to insure individuals for medical care or life who have inherited the probability of getting certain diseases? Will there be job discrimination, education discrimination, etc.? Instead of the current cultural, ethnic, and racial discrimination, a new form of "genetic" discrimination could occur. These are all things to be prepared for and to govern against by legislation.

PART 4

Nongenetic Risk Factors

"The mystique of science proclaims that numbers are the ultimate test of objectivity. Surely we can weigh a brain or score an intelligence test without recording our social preferences. If ranks are displayed in hard numbers obtained by rigorous and standardized procedures, then they must reflect reality. . . . If quantitative data are as subject to cultural constraint as any other aspect of science, then they have no special claim upon final truth."

—Steven Jay Gould, *The Mismeasure of Man*, 1981

Do birth complications cause schizophrenia?

Is schizophrenia more common in some cultural or racial groups than others?

Can bad family relationships cause schizophrenia?

More . . .

58. Do birth complications cause schizophrenia?

Numerous studies on the association of obstetric complications (both prenatal and perinatal) with schizophrenia have been reported over the years. No single specific complication has been implicated, however. These are a summation of various things, such as bleeding during pregnancy, influenza during the second trimester, premature birth, and excessively long labor. Some investigators have hypothesized that many birth complications lead to transient hypoxia to the developing brain, and when occurring at a particular stage in development, the fully developed brain will later be more vulnerable to schizophrenia. Particularly, it is thought that the cells of the **hippocampus** are most vulnerable to perinatal complications, such that its growth may be suppressed during a crucial time period. These are just theories without proof, and in fact, some good studies exist that now show no association of later schizophrenia with having been born with birth complications. At least one study of siblings with and without schizophrenia shows that they have no difference in frequency of birth complications. Thus, how can one draw conclusions about these data? First, the studies examining birth complications use various methods for selecting control individuals for comparison and for obtaining a history of birth complications. Controls need to be matched for social class and sex. When this is done by comparison to well siblings for an example, then the association with birth complications is less clear. Similarly, taking an obstetric history from mothers is fraught with bias, as it has been shown that mothers tend to remember more birth complications occurring in their chronically ill offspring than those who are well.

Hippocampus

This relatively small brain structure lies deep within the temporal lobe and is thought to be crucial for memory. It has been given this name because of its unusual shape.

Thus, the stronger studies are those that are prospective analyses of large birth cohorts where data have been archived systematically from birth. Several of these in the United Kingdom and United States have been published with equivocal results overall. Given that the vast majority of adults who have a history of having been born after prenatal complications *do not* develop schizophrenia, it is suspected that these are not significant risk factors for schizophrenia. Mothers who suffer such complications should not have to worry that in the future their offspring will be any more likely to develop schizophrenia than their peers. Pediatricians should not be warning of such.

59. Is schizophrenia more common in some cultural or racial groups than others?

The answer to this question most likely is *no.* Steven J. Gould, in his book *The Mismeasure of Man*, showed that seemingly objective quantitative data can be shown to be erroneously associated with the wrong characteristics due to societal bias, such as in the association of head size and intelligence (see the quote at the start of **Part 4**). Some studies have associated schizophrenia with lower socioeconomic status, and in some countries, this diagnosis appears more frequently in one racial or cultural group rather than another. The reasons for this are many. First, physicians tend to be more likely to diagnose schizophrenia rather than other forms of psychosis in persons who do not communicate well because their culture or language is different from the physician's or because it is not understood well. For example, in some religious sects in the United States and other countries, services become highly emotional with chanting that can give some people the appearance of being acutely psychotic, as people are "communicating with God." In some cultures, paranoia may be justified given the political history that some individuals may have encountered. The examples can go on. Nevertheless, the World Health Association has conducted multicenter incidence studies to show that schizophrenia is present throughout the world at relatively similar incidence rates across many different cultures. Other reports indicate its presence in Papua New Guinea (despite previous reports to the contrary), the Australian aboriginals, and the isolated ancient San population of South Africa. In fact, schizophrenia is possibly present in every population of the world because its origins are as old as the origins of modern *Homo sapiens* themselves. Schizophrenia has been described as "the price *Homo sapiens* pays for language," (Crow, 1997) meaning that schizophrenia is at the extreme of the uniquely human genetic variation that distinguishes modern human beings from all other primates and gave us the ability to communicate by complex language.

Nevertheless, there do exist many disparities in the diagnosis and treatment of schizophrenia across ethnic and racial groups. These are sensitive issues, but their underlying basis needs to be better understood. Rather than being fuel for stigmatizing groups, the differences, whether they be socially or biologically induced, need to be recognized so that each group may be better served with individualized treatments as needed.

60. Can bad family relationships cause schizophrenia?

An emphatic answer to this question is *no*, and this myth must be dispelled. Several years ago, it was popular among psychiatrists and psychologists to presume that the cause of schizophrenia had to do with poor mothering, or the "schizophrenogenic mother," as the term became coined. This was a mother that was supposedly giving mixed messages to her child, causing pathologic ambivalence and confusion. This notion, however, was not based on any carefully controlled research studies, but rather on subjective observations of some well-respected, psychodynamically oriented senior psychiatrists of the time. Another set of researchers introduced the term *expressed emotion* to the field and produced data to suggest that the greater the expressed emotion in a family, the more likely a psychosis would develop in an individual. These data, however, were refuted by others who argued that higher expressed emotion in *any* family with a schizophrenic member may have more to do with the frustration the family feels having to deal with a chronically ill individual who can cause frequent serious crises by virtue of the disorder itself. At best, one can say that a kind, reassuring, protective, and supportive intact family will aid someone afflicted with schizophrenia to have a better outcome to his or her illness than a disruptive and unsupportive family environment.

In the 1960s, the concept that schizophrenia was due to miscommunication among members of a nuclear family was very popular. Families were thought to be communicating in a strange way using what were called "double-binds" and "schisms" that only served to confuse the developing child. Of course, the mother, who had the most intense interaction with the child, was considered "schizophrenigenic" as mentioned above. A famous analyst, Frieda Fromm-Reichman, was known to espouse the theory of regressing patients back to infancy and then bringing the patient back to his or her current age with a particular kind of analysis that claimed to recreate the mothering that was never received. In addition, family therapy was given for the families of a patient with schizophrenia and the notion that one person was "the patient" was banned. Rather, the idea was that the whole family was "the patient" and that family therapy would resolve the symptoms that were appearing in one of its members. Unfortunately, this concept has caused much harm to families and their relationships with psychiatrists trying to treat the patient. Currently, no scientific basis suggests that a family's style of communication—and the mother's in particular—has had anything to do with the development of schizophrenia in any one individual.

61. Can immigration from another country increase risk for schizophrenia?

Some very interesting studies in the United Kingdom and the Netherlands have shown that Afro-Caribbean immigrants and other migrant groups to foreign countries have an increased incidence of schizophrenia in themselves and their offspring after having arrived in a foreign culture. Currently, the cause of this phenomenon is unclear—that is, whether it is genetic or environmental or an artifact of the data collection. However, the difficulties adjusting to life in a foreign country economically and socially can certainly provide fertile ground for the development of all kinds of emotional problems in later life. Despite these reports, the vast majority of immigrants to new lands do not develop schizophrenia. One could comment that countries such as the United States and Australia, in which the population is made up by a majority of different waves of immigrant groups over time, have not reported increases in schizophrenia as a result.

62. Does where you live affect your risk for illness (urban versus rural environments)?

Some epidemiologic surveys have found that schizophrenia appears more prevalent in urban than rural areas within the same country. Similarly, the prevalence of schizophrenia may be less, although the incidence the same, in underdeveloped rather than developed industrialized countries. This may be comparable to the urban versus rural distinction. Reasons for this disparity could be many but may have to do with the outcome of acute psychotic episodes. In general, rural and nonindustrialized societies tend to have extended families living together or close by, and thus emotional support for psychotic individuals is greater. These individuals also tend to be tolerated more in these environments and have more space to be alone so that they do not need to interact by force with others. It would be easier to stay out of a hospital or treatment facility existing in such environments. Recovery might be seen as a nonviolent, quiet behavior, and the inner world of someone with schizophrenia would not only be more tolerable but less noticeable. This does not mean, however, that it is better to live in a rural area if you have schizophrenia! Urban environments tend to provide patients with better medical care, more available psychiatrists and related healthcare personnel, and better access to the newest treatments.

63. Is schizophrenia infectious?

A Russian physician who reported the results from an epidemiological survey of dwellings in Moscow claimed that clusters of schizophrenia occurred in specific neighborhoods (Kasanetz, 1979). Torrey, in his book on *Schizophrenia and Civilization* (1980), claimed that pockets of schizophrenia exist in counties of Ireland, suggesting that schizophrenia could be infectious or spread from one individual to another. Crow and Done (1986), however, in a landmark analysis of a large number of pairs of siblings with schizophrenia, showed that despite two siblings living together having schizophrenia, the time of onset of their illness was not correlated, although their age of onset was. If an illness is contagious, one expects that two people living together would get it relatively close in time. If they seem to get the illness at the same age, the onset is predetermined by other factors such as developmental and/or genetic ones. Thus, the infectious theory "holds no water" and has largely been abandoned. However, environmental factors more prevalent in an urban environment could still be contributors, and this has not been ruled out.

64. Do viruses cause schizophrenia?

Dating back to Menninger in the early 1900s, there was a suspicion that viruses could cause schizophrenia. As Karl Menninger noted (1926), the great influenza epidemic of 1918 saw an increase of schizophrenia admissions to hospitals. Through the years since, particularly revived by Torrey and Peterson (1976), the viral hypothesis of schizophrenia has carried weight among some researchers even today. Many viral infections have been implicated besides influenza, such as cytomegalovirus, human herpesvirus I and II, Epstein-Barr virus, and some uniquely human retroviruses. The positive findings from these studies, however, have not been consistently replicated, and no active viral particles have ever been definitively isolated from the brains of people with schizophrenia after death. The most prevalent theory about these viruses is that a mother acquires the infection during the second trimester of pregnancy, a crucial time for brain higher cortical center development, and that this makes offspring more vulnerable to develop schizophrenia in later life. This is just a theory that does not yet produce convincing substantiating evidence.

PART 5

Substance Abuse and Schizophrenia

"It was very well to say 'Drink me,'" but the wise little Alice was not going to do that in a hurry. 'No, I'll look first,' she said, 'and see whether it is marked "poison" or not.'... However, this bottle was not marked 'poison,' so Alice ventured to taste it, and finding it very nice...very soon finished it off."

—Down the Rabbit-Hole, *Alice's Adventures in Wonderland,* by Lewis Carroll, 1865

Can the use of multiple street drugs in adolescence cause schizophrenia?

Can cannabis/marijuana specifically cause schizophrenia?

Can someone who has schizophrenia smoke cannabis/marijuana? Is it harmful, or can it also be beneficial?

More...

65. Can the use of multiple street drugs in adolescence cause schizophrenia?

It has long been known that various street drugs are used by people who develop an acute first episode of schizophrenia, and that patients and their families often blame the first episode on these drugs. Although there is an increased drug use in people developing schizophrenia compared with those who do not of similar ages, it has long been controversial as to which really comes first, drug abuse or schizophrenia. Can certain drugs cause schizophrenia, or does having subtle emotional signs of "pre-schizophrenia" cause people to alleviate their uncomfortable feelings or behaviors by experimenting with drugs? Alternatively, the use of drugs may simply bring on what is already an incipient illness faster.

Street drug use in general has been associated with an earlier age of onset of schizophrenia and with a poorer outcome, and it is particularly relevant to males with the illness, as males tend to abuse drugs significantly more than females. The kind of drug that can be harmful also depends on what is popular during a particular era and what is readily available. This, of course, varies geographically worldwide and with time.

Amphetamines

A category of drugs that sometimes are used illicitly under names such as "speed" or "ecstasy"; they tend to produce heightened arousal and are widely abused.

Cannabis

The herbaceous plant *Cannabis sativa* the leaves of which are often smoked or ingested to produce euphoria and relaxation. Use of cannabis has been linked with the onset of schizophrenia.

Various drugs that have been associated with schizophrenia-like symptoms were popular at different points in time and were also known by various street names, but they broadly include **amphetamines** (speed or ecstasy), methamphetamines, phencyclidine (PCP, angel dust), lysergic acid diethylamide (LSD), **cannabis** (marijuana or hash), cocaine (coke or crack), and opiates (heroin, morphine). LSD was "the" drug of the 1960s to the point that songs were popularized about its use. Cannabis remains the most frequently used drug among adolescents in the United States today. Unfortunately, if abused and used heavily, it has adverse consequences on their functioning regardless of whether it will lead to schizophrenia.

Some street drugs, such as methamphetamines and PCP, are known to mimic symptoms of schizophrenia acutely in otherwise normal people who are given doses of them, sometimes with long-term effects that persist even when the drugs are no longer taken. Both of these drugs are epidemic in some countries. Methamphetamine use is particularly high and widely prevalent in many South Asian and African countries, and thus psychiatrists in these countries are finding difficulty separating true chronic schizophrenia from continuous methamphetamine use.

However, other drugs of abuse, such as opiates and benzodiazepines are also commonly used by people with schizophrenia, as well as others who do not have schizophrenia. They are not known to cause schizophrenia, but their use is a problem of epidemic proportions and if someone with schizophrenia is also addicted to drugs and/or alcohol, they likely do not then comply with their prescribed treatments and tend to have a poor outcome and frequent relapses.

66. Can cannabis/marijuana specifically cause schizophrenia?

Numerous studies now show a strong association between marijuana use and the development of schizophrenia. Some believe that this newly reported association results from the substantial increase in potency of marijuana over recent years, which makes the marijuana now available on the streets considerably more potent than it was a few decades ago. Marijuana is also easily available compared with other street drugs. Thus, it would not be advisable for people already diagnosed with schizophrenia to use marijuana, nor should those with a known risk of the disease use it (e.g., relatives of a person with schizophrenia).

67. Can someone who has schizophrenia smoke cannabis/marijuana? Is it harmful, or can it also be beneficial?

In general, after schizophrenia is diagnosed, continued use of street sold cannabis or marijuana can only be harmful, because it reduces the likelihood of response to neuroleptic and other medications. In patients with schizophrenia, marijuana can produce reactions that are often not euphoric and calming, as in their peers who do not have schizophrenia, although the mechanism for this difference is not known. Use of marijuana also may produce a lack of compliance with oral medication by the patients, which leads to a poor outcome and rehospitalization, which may occur repeatedly until they realize the need to stay away from marijuana. Nevertheless, while in general cannabis use should be avoided by those with schizophrenia or related illnesses, some people who have had chronic schizophrenia for long periods of time claim that marijuana alleviates the very bothersome auditory hallucinations, and others get relief from general anxiety, particularly social anxiety when they are with other people. In fact, there is good evidence that the brain has receptors for cannabis compounds (called CB1 and CB2) and that compounds that these receptors function abnormally in people with schizophrenia. Thus, some of the compounds present in cannabis may modulate them in some way that does provide relief from symptoms. However, the plant we know as marijuana or cannabis (*Cannabis sativa*) is made up of over 400 different compounds. The one considered to be its active ingredient that gives the effects people using it like is tetrahydrocannabinol (THC). One of the other major compounds, cannabidiol (CBD), is thought to be beneficial for schizophrenia. The problem is that marijuana bought on the street has varying proportions of the different active ingredients from the cannabis plant, and different varieties or subspecies of the *Cannabis sativa* plant itself may have innately different amounts of each compound. In some states in the U.S. and also countries in Europe where marijuana has been legalized (whether for medical or personal use), businesses have sprung up that are manufacturing and purifying the active ingredients of the cannabis plant to give different effects. Drugs derived from these compounds that are in treatment trials currently for neurological disorders, such as epilepsy, multiple sclerosis, and chronic pain disorders such as fibromyalgia, may soon be in trials as well for psychiatric symptoms such as general anxiety, sleep disorders, and even schizophrenia. There has already been one small trial in post-traumatic stress disorder (PTSD) showing beneficial effects on symptoms such as nightmares, although larger and more trials need to be performed. The current group of cannabis-derived manufactured medications are called dronabinol (Marinol®), nabilone (Cesamet®), and nabiximols (Sativex®).

68. Which drugs cause schizophrenia-like symptoms in people who do not have schizophrenia?

All hallucinogens, particularly LSD and PCP, and the many amphetamine compounds can cause schizophrenia-like symptoms in normal individuals, but these symptoms clear up once the drug is removed from one's blood circulation. In most instances, the individual has a complete recovery in a matter of minutes or hours. However, sometimes these compounds can leave lasting effects long after they have been eliminated (days to months), and the individual will then likely visit a hospital emergency room. Urine screens may be able to detect which drug classes have been used, but not always. (See Question 65.)

69. What does drug use do to people who have schizophrenia?

It is widely known that people who frequently use street drugs when they have schizophrenia not only have negative effects from the drugs that people without schizophrenia do not have, but in general they have a poorer outcome. They do not function well in the community, have more negative symptoms, and have persistence of their positive symptoms. This may be due to noncompliance with medication and other treatment regimes as well as possible interaction of the antipsychotic medications with the street drugs themselves. Patients who continue to use street drugs should be treated with dual-diagnosis therapies that give them options and motivation to terminate use of such drugs.

70. Can someone who has schizophrenia drink alcohol?

The simple answer is *no*. Alcohol, even in moderate amounts, precipitates affective symptoms, exacerbates the symptoms of schizophrenia, and usually leads to noncompliance with a medication regime and rehospitalization in many people. It also has adverse effects on blood levels of medications and can be particularly toxic to the liver when used in combination with any medications that are metabolized through the liver (which includes many "atypical" antipsychotics and clozapine). Regular alcohol use is certainly not advised, given that it is not easily used in careful moderation. An occasional beer on a social occasion for someone with schizophrenia, however, may be beneficial if it affords a way of socializing and meeting with peers—that is, becoming more integrated into everyday life. However, excessive or regular alcohol use is harmful to anyone, and those with schizophrenia are particularly sensitive.

71. Why do people with schizophrenia smoke cigarettes excessively?

It has long been noticed that patients on psychiatric hospital wards are almost all chain-smokers of cigarette, and numerous scientific surveys now confirm the association of cigarette smoking with schizophrenia. Behavioral therapies in the past were geared toward positive reinforcement by the attainment of a goal and thus "winning" a pack of cigarettes. You might think that the consequence of this would be that lung cancer and other cigarette-associated cancers would also be increased in schizophrenic patients, but this does not appear to be true. Whether people with schizophrenia smoke cigarettes so heavily because of their underlying psychopathology or because of a social consequence of having this illness is presently unclear. It may simply be that these people develop the addictive habit of cigarette smoking because of a need to occupy their hands and stimulate themselves with some oral gratification during times that are continually stressful and uncomfortable. However, this phenomenon has been noted to have a specific scientific basis by a well-known researcher in Colorado, Dr. Robert Freedman, who claimed that cigarette smoking, in essence a craving for nicotine, is so excessive among these patients because of an underlying abnormality in receptors for nicotine in the brain. His laboratory, and now many others, studied nicotine receptors in people with schizophrenia, the genetic susceptibility for abnormalities in these receptors and addiction to nicotine. One possibility is that the genetic abnormality that leads to nicotine addiction may somehow be related to a genetic risk for schizophrenia. Pharmaceutical companies are thus trying to identify some novel drugs that might counteract the nicotine receptor abnormalities and thus be efficacious in alleviating symptoms of schizophrenia. However, none have yet been found to be useful.

PART 6

The Biology Underlying Schizophrenia: Current Research Findings

"I think you have to speculate. If I have a good idea, I tend to believe it is true. An idea is better than no idea . . . that's the way good science works. An idea can be tested, whereas if you have no idea, nothing can be tested and you don't understand anything!"

—James D. Watson, interview published in *New York Times*, on the 50th Anniversary of the discovery of DNA, February 3, 2002

Are there any tests that can be taken from blood, urine, or spinal fluid to definitively diagnose schizophrenia?

Is schizophrenia a "chemical imbalance"?

Are there any differences in the brains of people who have schizophrenia?

More . . .

72. Are there any tests that can be taken from blood, urine, or spinal fluid to definitively diagnose schizophrenia?

Biological psychiatrists have been speculating about the causes of schizophrenia for a century and hypothesizing that various compounds, neuronal pathways, and brain structures may be involved. However, most of these speculations have led nowhere, and to date, unlike most other medical diseases, there are no blood, urine, or spinal fluid tests for this illness yet. You can find high blood sugar in diabetes or elevated **immunoglobulins** in multiple sclerosis, but nothing in schizophrenia, at least that holds up over time.

Immunoglobulins

The proteins that help the body respond to foreign substances and infections.

There have been plenty of good ideas brought forward and several hypotheses have been explored over the years. Many factors were found in 24-hour urine collections, serum, and spinal fluid. The notorious "pink spot" from the 1960s and '70s, a supposed litmus test for schizophrenia, was nothing other than metabolites of tea that the patients were drinking in excess. The so-called endogenous hallucinogens, chemicals produced in excess by one's own body, such as dimethyltryptamine and phenylethylamine, both turned out also to be artifactual findings, the former being caused by a laboratory method that had not been validated and the latter caused by nonspecific anxiety. Researchers have long abandoned the idea of looking for such factors; as we now know, the biology of schizophrenia is not that simple.

73. Is schizophrenia a "chemical imbalance"?

Many people speak of schizophrenia as a "chemical imbalance," which makes sense given that the medications that alleviate many symptoms are chemicals. What this actually *means*, however, is still not clear in research studies, and how the chemistry interacts with the structural brain changes is not known.

Many biochemical hypotheses about schizophrenia were formulated after neuroleptic medications were introduced. These drugs act directly on dopamine receptors, as well as other receptors, and their efficacy could specifically be shown to be directly related to dopamine activity by laboratory assays. Consequently, the dopamine hypothesis has always been the most prominent. In support of the dopamine hypothesis are studies showing that dopamine receptors measured in postmortem brain and also in **positron emission tomography** (**PET**) scans were elevated in patients with schizophrenia. Some evidence showed that these findings were not due to an effect of the medication, but rather the pathology of the illness itself. Serotonin, another brain neurotransmitter, as well as GABA and others, has been thought to be related somehow to schizophrenia pathology, likely by their effects on dopamine receptors.

Positron Emission Tomography (PET)

This is a radiologic procedure that measures the metabolism of a radiolabeled substance that is injected into a subject's vein and one that is known to enter the brain relatively rapidly. Pictures are then taken of the brain with the regions metabolizing the injected substance "lighting-up".

More recently, the "glutamate hypothesis" has become even more prominent than the dopamine hypothesis. L-glutamic acid (glutamate) is a major excitatory amino acid neurotransmitter throughout the brain and nervous system, and it is known that glutamate plays a major role in brain development, affecting neuronal migration, neuronal differentiation, axon genesis, and neuronal survival. It first was thought to be involved in schizophrenia; the popular recreational drug phencyclidine (PCP) was recognized to not only mimic schizophrenia in its actions, but also to exert its actions primarily on glutamate receptors. Several lines of evidence then suggested that a dysfunction in glutamatergic neurotransmission via the N-methyl-d-aspartate (NMDA) subtype of glutamate receptors might be involved in the pathophysiology of schizophrenia, and the NMDA receptor hypofunction hypothesis of schizophrenia became known. The dopamine hypothesis attributes hyperdopaminergic function as a possible cause of schizophrenia, whereas the glutamate hypothesis proposes a hypofunctional glutamate system. There is substantial evidence for both hypotheses, based on observations that certain classes of street drugs can produce schizophrenia-like symptoms in normal individuals. Not only does PCP produce symptoms most similar to schizophrenia by antagonizing the action of glutamate, but amphetamines also produce some of the acute positive symptoms by stimulating dopamine receptors. In general, PCP and similar drugs produce somewhat more of the positive and negative symptoms of schizophrenia than the amphetamine-like drugs. The latter fail to produce some of the core symptoms of schizophrenia, such as formal thought disorder and negative symptoms, although PCP may. Currently, initiated by the glutamate hypothesis, glycine and d-serine, both NMDA receptor stimulators, are being used as add-on medications to treat patients with chronic schizophrenia who do not completely benefit from other medications.

Most recently, some pharmaceutical companies have developed new agents that target the glutamate pathway by binding to one of its receptors. Some initial trials have shown modest improvement in the symptoms of schizophrenia using these drugs, but more trials will need to be done before these drugs are ready for FDA approval, and toxicity will have to be carefully evaluated.

74. *Are there any differences in the brains of people who have schizophrenia?*

The answer to this question is *yes*, but in a subtle way, and no finding is specific to the illness—nor is any one finding present in all patients with schizophrenia. Someone with schizophrenia could also have a completely normal brain. Since the beginning of the recognition of the concept of "dementia praecox," Kraepelin (1907) felt that this was a progressive brain disease, and he noted in his textbook that

> "*the course is progressive without remissions... Signs of mental deterioration may appear within a few months, and are usually well marked by the end of two years... On the other hand, there are some cases... which do not dement for a number of years.*" He also said early on (Kraepelin, 1899) that "*in view of the clinical and anatomical facts known so far I cannot doubt we are dealing with serious... and only partially reversible damage to the* **cerebral cortex**... *75 percent of cases reach higher grades of dementia and sink deeper and deeper.*"

By the time he published his 1919 text, Kraepelin illustrated what he thought was wrong in the brain with drawings of neurons that he described as "diseased with lipoid products of disintegration." Where his notions about the brain came from, however, are unclear, as there are no careful research studies that he or anyone else published to provide evidence for these claims.

By the 1930s, the technique of examining the brain by **pneumoencephalography**, a quite risky procedure of injecting air into the **ventricles** (the space that holds the cerebral spinal fluid that bathes the brain) in order to observe their outline, was applied to studies of patients

Cortex (cerebral cortex)

The outer portion of the brain. It consists mostly of the "gray matter" that contains nerve cells.

Pneumoencephalography

An X-ray picture of the brain taken by replacement of the cerebrospinal fluid with air or gas. This was a method used to detect whether a patient had brain atrophy prior to the invention of computed tomography and magnetic resonance imaging. This method is no longer in use.

Ventricles

As this term applies to the brain, the spaces connecting throughout the brain that provide a system for the circulation of the fluid present in the brain called cerebrospinal fluid.

with schizophrenia. Many reports showed enlargement of the ventricular space in chronic schizophrenia, clearly suggestive of atrophy of the brain at an age when this should not have been present. These results went quite unnoticed by most psychiatrists in the mid 20th century, probably because of the rise in psychological and psychoanalytic theories and approaches to schizophrenia. When biological psychiatry again became in vogue and new methods to examine the brain *in vivo* were developed, namely **computed tomography (CT)**, some important findings emerged. In 1976, a very small study of severely ill patients with chronic schizophrenia was published in the medical journal *The Lancet* (Johnstone et al., 1976). It clearly showed by CT that the patients had significantly larger brain ventricular size than age-matched controls. Soon many other investigators, using much larger, more representative samples of patients, widely replicated this finding. To date, this is probably the most replicated finding in all of schizophrenia research!

Computed tomography (CT)

A form of X-ray that is able to view the brain in more detail than a standard skull X-ray. The advantage CT has over MRI is that it detects bone change, whereas MRI views the brain tissue, and is not sensitive to bone.

Magnetic resonance imaging (MRI)

A method to examine the tissue of the brain using a magnetic field and computer system. The machine itself consists of a horizontal tube inside of a giant magnet. The patient having an MRI scan lies on his or her back and slides into the tube on a special table. After inside, the patient is scanned.

Gray matter

The brownish gray nerve tissue of the brain and spinal cord that contains the nerve cells.

White matter

Whitish brain and spinal cord tissue composed mostly of nerve fibers and its shiny protective coat called myelin.

In the late 1980s, brain-imaging methods produced even better direct anatomical windows into the *in vivo* brain with the advent of **magnetic resonance imaging (MRI)** scanners. The first studies, however, were performed using brain image "slices" that were very thick, so subtle changes that occur in small brain structures, or just subtle differences in general, could be easily missed. Over the decade that followed, however, MRI scanning became more and more refined, and brain images in living patients came to be seen in almost as much detail and contrast as direct postmortem brain visualization. MRI scanning currently is the main imaging technique used to evaluate the brains of people with schizophrenia. In MRI scans, the actual brain tissue, divided into **gray matter** containing the neuronal cells and **white matter** containing their fibrous connections, is clearly distinguishable.

As a result, a number of studies have shown various differences in the brains of patients with schizophrenia. These mostly include volume of structures. Besides the ventricles, the volume of gray matter as a whole is significantly less, as is the size of the temporal lobe and its different subdivisions (i.e., **superior temporal gyrus** and hippocampus), frontal lobe, and corpus callosum (**Table 2**) (**Figure 5**). We now know that there are also white matter changes in these structures.

Superior temporal gyrus
A portion of the temporal lobe of the brain that has many functions related to language, including understanding it.

Table 2 Brain Structures that Relate to Schizophrenia

Brain Structure	Function	Finding in Schizophrenia	Does the Finding Become Greater Over Time?	Comments
Ventricles	Holds spinal fluid that bathes the brain	Enlarged	Yes	Large ventricles mean that the brain tissue surrounding it is less than it should be
Frontal lobes	• Attention • Sequential planning • Processing new memory • Speaking • Some uniquely human mentalizing	Reduced gray matter	Unknown	This structure is difficult to measure, but its functioning has been shown in many ways to be abnormal
Temporal lobes	Auditory processing	Reduced volume	Possibly for all	
Superior temporal gyrus	Language	Reduced volume		
Hippocampus	Memory	Reduced volume		

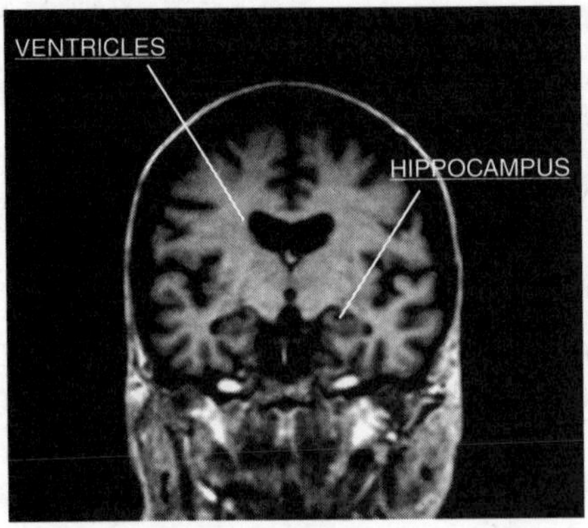

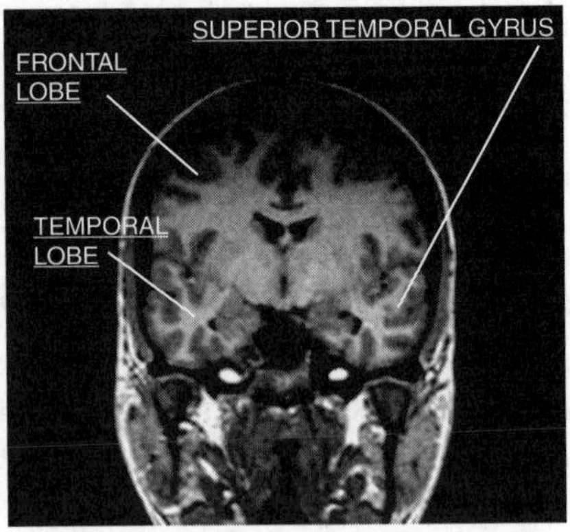

Figure 5 (1) MRI — Patient with schizophrenia (2) MRI — Normal patient

75. Should an MRI scan be performed?

In a clinical setting, a good evaluation of someone who is first being diagnosed with schizophrenia should include an MRI so that a baseline initial brain assessment is available for comparison in later years. It should also be used in people with characteristic symptoms of schizophrenia to exclude any other brain diseases, no matter how rare they are, that could mimic the symptoms of schizophrenia, such as temporal lobe tumors or any other known neurodegenerative disorder. The status of brain structural and functional findings could be helpful for considering what the likely outcome of an episode might be. It should also be performed on people who are considered in the prodromal stage of illness for predicting if conversion to full schizophrenia is imminent. If such is the case, early treatment may be beneficial for preventing further deterioration.

76. *Are functional MRI scans useful?*

Some other types of MRI scans that can be performed are **functional MRI (fMRI)** or **magnetic resonance spectroscopy** (MRS). In fMRI, subjects are given a task to perform that uses different brain anatomical regions while the scanner takes pictures of their brain. In patients with schizophrenia, the tasks usually include some type of behavior that requires a short period of memory or language detection by responding when hearing or seeing instructions. In general, the functioning of different parts of the brain is measurable by the intensity of activity in the working regions. Schizophrenia patients have been shown to have less focused and less lateralized functioning when responding to these tasks, although these studies are just initial research findings. More needs to be done before this kind of scanning can be applied to clinical situations.

Functional MRI (fMRI)

A brain scan that shows chemical actions taking place in the brain in response to a stimulus. The stimulus could be anything, such as voluntary movement of the fingers to memorizing a set of words.

Magnetic resonance spectroscopy (MRS)

A type of MRI scan that examines chemical spectras in the brain. These chemicals are those that are present in the structure of membranes or metabolic activity in nerve cells and between cells.

Similarly, MRS (magnetic resonance spectroscopy) is a quantitative imaging method to detect levels of neurochemicals in the brain in different regions. Abnormal amounts of these substances are thought to indicate evidence of brain disease at the biochemical level. These scans too, however, are not applicable to a clinical setting and thus far have only been research tools that present some complicated problems in their interpretation. Thus at present, neither fMRI or MRS are types of scans that are yet ready for the clinic. Neither are positron emission tomography (PET) scans, a more invasive procedure that is more useful in the detection of tumors and other neurodegenerative diseases, but not schizophrenia.

77. Should an EEG be done on patients with schizophrenia?

Electroencephalogram (EEG)

A type of test whereby electrodes are placed on several areas of the head and recordings are made of the brain electrical activity.

Certain findings in **electroencephalogram (EEG)** scans are characteristic of people with schizophrenia. For example, some of the EEG brain waves that are produced when the subject is stimulated in some way are known as "evoked potentials" or "event-related potentials (ERPs)." There are many terms used for observations in EEGs that appear relevant to schizophrenia and are worth noting because they have been associated with underlying neurotransmitter or the biochemical abnormalities noted above and also may be predictive of people who are at high risk for developing schizophrenia. One is called mismatch negativity, which is a response to an aberrant tone in a series of consistent ones. Patients with schizophrenia have reduced amplitudes of the EEG waves associated with this response, particularly over the frontal and temporal lobes, when they are stimulated with an odd sound or visual object. Two other wave components measured in schizophrenia and found to be abnormal are the p300 and the p50. The p300 wave component is evaluated during a decision-making task, such as making a decision about two different flashed numbers or sounds, particularly when an odd or deviant one is identified among many usual ones. The p50 is considered a measure of sensory gating, whereby the brain "tunes out" a second sound that occurs after a first one. Both the p300 and the p50 have been found to be abnormal when measured in people with schizophrenia. Another physiological phenomenon, the prepulse-inhibition response, is when a weaker stimulus inhibits a response to a much stronger one, such as the startle response. This is measured, not by the EEG electrodes, but by a different apparatus with a few electrodes that can measure skin and/or eyelid response. Patients with schizophrenia are deficient in this response.

These tests might also be worth conducting because they are associated with other symptoms, such as cognitive ones, and similar to the MRI, may be able to give some prognostic indication. However, for the most part, they are still considered research tools and not available in a clinical setting. The EEG would, however, certainly be useful clinically if a seizure disorder were suspected.

78. When do the brain changes occur, and is schizophrenia considered a progressive brain disorder?

Patients with chronic schizophrenia are known to have recognizable changes in brain structures as mentioned in Question 74, but *when* they begin to become abnormal in the lifetime of an individual is still controversial. Studies of patients at the first episode, however, are able to detect many of the changes, suggesting that they may occur even before the illness is noticeable. There is some evidence from a couple of recent studies of high-risk individuals that the brain changes actually do predate illness and the brain continues to deteriorate along with the development of symptoms. There is also now evidence from several studies following patients after their first episode of illness that suggest that the brain continues to change at a more rapid rate than that of the normal aging process. Brain tissue seems to be lost at a greater rate over time sporadically throughout the illness (see **Figure 6**). A lot of publicity has also been given to a few researchers who have provided data that show that neuroleptic medication may cause changes over time in brain stuctures, such that it would be possible that the progressive change seen could be related to medications. It is unlikely, however, that this could be the explanation, since brain structural changes were occuring prior to the use of neuroleptic medications and studies in people who have never been treated also show the characteristic brain changes. Nevertheless, this is currently an open debated question. Similarly, some studies show that the tissue loss seems to be correlated to the severity of illness, while others do not. This effect is difficult to separate from the effect of medications, since the more severe the illness, the more likely the patient is to receive more and higher doses of medications. Even if some tissue loss is due to a lifetime of taking medications that affect brain structure and its functioning, it is not clear that this is a bad thing, nor is it likely to be the only explanation for progressive brain change in schizophrenia.

More research is needed on this topic, but its implications are vast: If there is progressive brain structural change characteristic of schizophrenia and it is related to the evolution of clinical symptoms, then medications need to be given early to prevent progression. Several research groups are now working on this issue and hopefully will soon produce recommendations about early treatment and the types of treatment. Table 2 outlines the changes that have been found in brains of patients with schizophrenia and whether there is evidence of progressive change in these structures. Figure 6 illustrates an example of one such case of a young 34-year-old female with schizophrenia whose ventricles appear to have consistently enlarged over time from her first episode of illness to 5 and then 10 years later.

For over a decade, most investigators have thought that the brain structural abnormalities of schizophrenia must at least in part be neurodevelopmental in origin—that is, occurring either because of an insult prenatally to the developing brain or because of a neuronal growth defect prenatally that is perhaps genetically controlled. One alternative hypothesis was that in adolescent-onset illness, the reorganization of brain connections during that time might be occurring abnormally. The reasons for constructing these theories as an alternative to thinking of schizophrenia as a progressive, degenerative process mainly were that the length of illness duration could never be correlated with the amount of abnormal brain change and that no cellular signs of degeneration have ever been shown in brains of patients with schizophrenia. It has now become clear, however, from results of carefully conducted longitudinal studies that brain ventricular size continues to expand over time and that none of the anomalies associated with schizophrenia appear static, whether or not they begin early in development. (See Figure 4 in **Part 4**, “Genetic Risk,” for a combination of both the neurodevelopmental and degenerative hypotheses.)

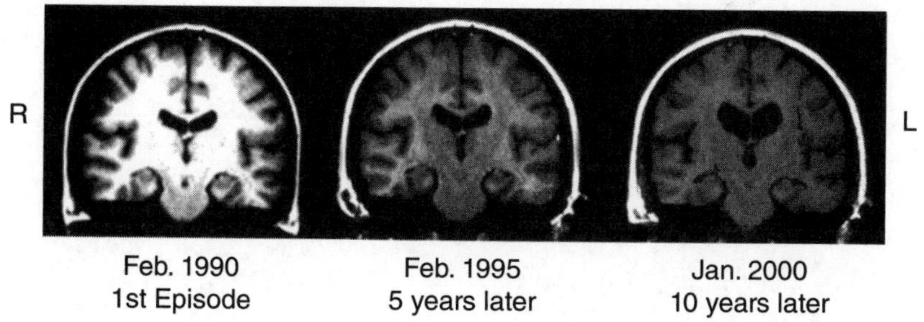

Figure 6 Ten-year MRI follow-up in a 34-year-old female with chronic schizophrenia.

79. Could the brain changes be due to an inflammatory process?

Many years ago, antibody levels were studied in patients with chronic schizophrenia, and one hypothesis was that schizophrenia could be due to an autoantibody response to one's own cells, particularly in the brain. However, despite elevations of anti-brain antibodies and various other indicators of autoimmunity, eventually it was thought that these findings were related to long-term treatment with medications and not a primary immune disorder.

Recently, however, renewed interest in this phenomenon has been getting attention. Patients at the beginning of illness have been reported with elevated blood levels of several immune-response indicators called cytokines, and also elevated blood levels of the hormone cortisol, an indicator of response to stress. Other studies have shown brain evidence of proliferation of glial cells, tissue indicators of an inflammatory response. At this point in time, however, it is unclear whether this process could be a marker for illness onset and primary to the illness pathology. If it is, then new drugs targeting the inflammatory response might be useful to prevent some of the brain changes described here.

PART 7

Violence and Aggression in Schizophrenia

"Is this a dagger I see before me, The handle toward my hand? Come, let me clutch thee,. . . . I go, and it is done. The bell invites me. Hear it not, Duncan; for it is a knell That summons thee to heaven or to hell."

—Shakespeare, *Macbeth*, Act 2, Scene 1

Do people with schizophrenia frequently commit violent acts and crimes?

What should I do if my relative or friend is behaving violently or expressing violent thoughts?

How can violent behavior be predicted?

More . . .

80. Do people with schizophrenia frequently commit violent acts and crimes?

Violence is *not* a symptom of schizophrenia. An individual with schizophrenia is not more dangerous than any other person, provided that he or she is treated with medication for symptoms. In fact, people with schizophrenia are far more likely to harm themselves than others.

However, there is a conception that people with schizophrenia are violent by nature of the illness itself. This notion is likely to be based particularly on cases that gain a lot of publicity and are subjects of movies. Notable cases include the paranoid schizophrenia patient who was released from a Long Island, New York, state psychiatric hospital many years ago, convincing his physician that he no longer had the delusion that his estranged wife must die, only to immediately go to her home and murder her, or the hallucinating homeless man who pushed a young girl onto the New York City subway track and into the path of an incoming train. Ted Kaczynski, the "Unabomber," was clearly suffering from paranoid schizophrenia and a thought disorder that was certainly evident in the manifesto he sent to *The New York Times*. In the United Kingdom, a serial killer known as the "Yorkshire Ripper," suffered from schizophrenia and was committed to a long-stay psychiatric forensic hospital after his trial. The man with severe paranoia who shot many random people on the Long Island Railroad certainly had all the signs of untreated paranoid schizophrenia for years, but most people did not pay enough attention to getting him to treatment. Another famous case was the young man, John Hinckley, Jr., who felt the delusional need to shoot President Reagan many years ago; he was diagnosed with schizophrenia and has spent many years since in a psychiatric hospital. More recently there have been several other cases, such as the young man who killed several people in a Colorado movie theatre, or the individual who shot a congresswoman in the head, killing others while she was about to give a public speech, and the case of the troubled young man who killed his mother and then dozens of school children and teachers in Connecticut.

These cases were *all* individuals who were either not diagnosed or were not maintained on medications and had evolving illness that spiraled out of control before healthcare professionals could intervene. In several cases, the affected individual had a long history of unstable behavior and several warning signs of psychopathological behavior that, had they known what to look for, would have led family, friends, and professionals to intervene much earlier. However, at the present, we really have no strong predictors of who will or will not become violent, prior to a first recognizable episode of schizophrenia, except for a prior history of violence itself. In the famous case of John Hinckley, over the years prior to his crime, he became obsessed with the movie *Taxi Driver*, which was about an American psychopath who stalks the president of the United States. Jodie Foster, the actress who played an attractive young woman in the movie, was the focus of his delusion; Hinckley saw himself becoming romantically involved with to the point of stalking her with letters and attempted visits while she was a student at Yale. Some people say that his obsession with this movie (whose chief character stalks a president) is what drove him to purchase handguns and eventually on March 29, 1981, to shoot and wound President Reagan and his press secretary James Brady, as well as two other individuals on the scene. He was tried and eventually found not guilty by reason of insanity and sent to the special forensic unit at St. Elizabeth's Hospital in Washington, DC. The tragedy is that if *any* of the professionals, including psychiatrists, whom he had seen during the several years preceding this event had identified the correct diagnosis and treated him effectively with neuroleptic medication, the violence he inflicted on the president and others would likely not have occurred.

In Boston a few years ago, there was the tragic case of the so-called "Craigslist Killer." The person alleged to have committed this crime was a star medical student who was liked by all and not suspected of having any mental illness, yet the bizarre story of how he browsed through the erotic section of Craigslist to find women who were offering massage and other sexually provocative services and then murdered one is similar to the Yorkshire Ripper in many ways. He, too, was likely suffering from an underlying undetected psychosis, although we will never be sure, as he eventually committed suicide while in jail awaiting trial. Thus, many such stories give the public the impression that people with schizophrenia, by virtue of their diagnosis, are dangerous.

Despite some of the previous examples, when violence does occur, it is not premeditated and is most frequently targeted at family members. In addition, all these examples of violent crimes were committed when the perpetrator was in an unstable stage of illness that was untreated. The subway incident described previously here was the stimulus for New York State to pass a mandatory outpatient treatment law (Kendra's Law, named after the girl who was pushed onto the subway tracks and died) so that patients with schizophrenia who are released from hospitals cannot voluntarily choose to discontinue their medications. Several other states now have similar laws.

Criminal behavior is not just limited to acts of violence. Various other crimes, such as robbery, property damage, and many infractions of the law, can lead to jail sentences. Antisocial behavior, commonly known as psychopathy, is clearly associated with crime, but large studies of individuals with and without schizophrenia suggest that having schizophrenia does not necessarily mean the patient has a psychopathy. On the other hand, regardless of whether an individual has a psychotic diagnosis, the presence of psychopathy is associated with criminal behavior. In addition, family studies do not show an excess clustering of psychopathy among relatives of schizophrenic patients, indicating that this behavior is not genetically associated with schizophrenia. So, in summary, most people with schizophrenia are not psychopaths, and most psychopaths do not have schizophrenia—and it is the psychopath who is more likely to commit crimes. In individuals with schizophrenia like those described above who do engage in criminal acts or violence, it is almost always due to lack of treatment or an effective treatment that alleviates their symptoms.

81. What should I do if my relative or friend is behaving violently or expressing violent thoughts?

Many people close to patients with schizophrenia are frustrated with the mental healthcare system as it currently exists in the United States, because in most instances it does not provide support for a sick individual until he or she is already an immediate threat to others or acutely threatening suicide. In these circumstances, of course, the police emergency phone number should be called immediately, and the patient must be subdued and brought to a psychiatric hospital. Unfortunately, these patients are too often victims of accidental violence by frightened police officers, who then provide severe force to suppress the violent individuals and in some cases inflict injuries and even death. Police forces and all types of public emergency response personnel must be trained in the acute care of these individuals and how to safely transport them to psychiatric emergency rooms. Too often, patients are instead brought to jail and kept there for many days without much-needed medications. Families and friends can be instrumental support at times like these to ensure that patients receive the proper treatment and legal representation.

82. How can violent behavior be predicted?

The likelihood of violence is increased by alcohol or street drug intake. Patients who are noncompliant with a prescribed medication regime can then become violent. The most important predictor of violent behavior is a past history of violence, whether or not someone has schizophrenia. Strong predictors of violence in the mentally ill are the feeling that others are out to harm one's self and the feeling that one's mind is dominated by forces beyond ones control or that thoughts are being put into one's head.

Another symptom that may predict violence is a specific type of hallucination called "command hallucinations," in which internal voices are heard as if they were coming from the outside telling the individual what to do and in many cases to either harm oneself or someone else. The presence of this type of hallucination and the need to act on it may be a compelling predictor of violence.

Often, however, police pick up individuals with schizophrenia in general as a precautionary measure because they do not know when someone who is behaving out of the ordinary is likely to be violent. Such is especially true in Washington, DC, where caution may be essential but can sometimes be an overreaction. For example, it is common for many people with paranoid or other types of schizophrenia from all over the country to travel to the nation's capital to address their many delusions about the FBI, the Internal Revenue Service, or even the president. At St. Elizabeth's Hospital, once a Federal Psychiatric Institution in the late 20th century, a special ward existed for many years in the forensic division for the "White House cases." Anyone who threatened the president would be brought there and could not be released until the Secret Service allowed it. On one occasion, I evaluated a patient on this ward whose only crime was feeling that he had many things in common with then-president Gerald Ford and simply presented himself at the gate of the White House requesting to "share his bubble gum with President Ford!"

Education of law enforcement officers, the Secret Service, and the FBI in how to diffuse violent behavior and how to manage patients with schizophrenia is essential.

PART 8

Suicidal Behavior and Schizophrenia

"They heard her singing her last song,
The Lady of Shalott....
Till her blood was frozen slowly,
And her eyes were darkened wholly....
Who is this? And what is here?
And in the lighted palace near
Died the sound of royal cheer...
But Lancelot mused a little space;
He said, "She has a lovely face;
God in his mercy lend her grace,
The Lady of Shalott."

—Alfred Lord Tennyson,
"The Lady of Shalott," Part IV

What are the signs of suicidal thoughts in schizophrenia?

What can be done to prevent suicide attempts?

More...

83. What are the signs of suicidal thoughts in schizophrenia?

It is commonly thought that suicide is solely a characteristic of depression, but this is not so. Approximately 1 in 10 people with schizophrenia commit suicide. The average lifespan of people with schizophrenia is less than that of the general population, and this may partially be due to suicide. Suicide attempts are several-fold more common than the suicides that are successfully completed.

The most vulnerable period for suicide is when most people with this diagnosis are young, newly diagnosed, treated with medications for the first time, and recently discharged from the hospital. Often these individuals have not been properly connected to supportive networks and regular treatment. They have also not been adequately educated about their illness and the need for continual medication, or they were denying that the healthcare professionals were correct. Frequently, they believe that after the symptoms have subsided, they will be back to their **premorbid** state, and thus they can discontinue any medication recommended. However, they find it difficult to adjust to their old lives and return to the independence that they enjoyed before becoming ill. Many friends have deserted them, and a general lack of connection and closeness to other people results. This is a period when strong support, guidance, and frequent professional observation and follow-up are needed.

Premorbid

The time period before any symptoms of a disorder, including subtle signs, have developed.

In addition, being unmarried, coming from a high socioeconomic family background, and having high intelligence and high life expectations all lead to a feeling of loss, hopelessness, and isolation. If the individual then does not comply with the prescribed treatments and turns to street drugs, the suicidal risk increases substantially. With regard to symptoms that are likely to lead to suicide, depression is by far the most common among individuals with schizophrenia, as it is in all cases of suicide. In contrast to public understanding, depression is present in the majority of people with schizophrenia at some time during the course of their illness. Less frequently present are the paranoid attacks of panic that lead to suicidal acts and provide the only way out of the delusion of being chased or followed. Occasionally, patients who attempt suicide are responding to voices commanding them to harm themselves.

Sometimes patients have suicidal thoughts (in addition to suicide attempts) because they see their futures as overwhelming and with nothing left but a lifelong continuance of the painful symptoms they describe, as well as never being able to discontinue taking the medications that produce side effects. Support from family, friends, and therapists is essential to give these patients hope for a good quality of life in the future.

In the book *Night Falls Fast*, Kay Jamison describes the development of psychotic and depressive behavior in a close friend that eventually led him to commit suicide. She struggled with the question, could this have been prevented if she had been there for him? This was one of the reflections that she will never be able to answer. The book, however, clearly describes all the signs of impending suicide and how one may survive them, as she herself did. Suicide is the ultimate way that people with schizophrenia deal with their struggles with thoughts and hallucinations they cannot control. These cause pain as clearly as physical injuries can. They may eventually commit suicide because of the "pain" and thus, the subtitle of this book is "Painful Minds."

84. What can be done to prevent suicide attempts?

The foremost important prevention measure is to provide intensive frequent follow-up for newly diagnosed patients. Support systems must be in place before release of such patients from the hospital, and these must include not only psychiatric care but also occupational rehabilitation, family support, social support, financial support, and then finally, follow-up by healthcare personnel to make sure that a comprehensive treatment plan occurs. It is now thought that certain medications may be particularly beneficial and protective against suicidal thoughts, although the mechanism for this action is not clearly understood. One such medication that has been shown in a large trial to lead to significantly less suicidal behavior than other medications is clozapine (see Question 32). This effect may be due to clozapine's prominent stimulant action on serotonin receptors in the brain, although this is only a theory. Suicide has long been associated with low brain levels of the metabolites of serotonin and may indicate low serotonergic tone in the brain. Serotonin is a neurotransmitter that is abundant in brain regions that are associated with emotion. It is thus possible that low moods are a reflection of low serotonin, which is supported by the knowledge that newer antidepressants called the serotonin receptor uptake inhibitors (SSRIs) raise the availability of serotonin in brain tissue and are helpful in alleviating depression whether or not depression is the primary diagnosis.

PART 9

Issues for Women

"The day will come when men will recognize woman as his peer, not only at the fireside, but in councils of the nation. Then, and not until then, will there be a perfect comradeship, the ideal union between the sexes that will result in the highest development of the race."

—Susan B. Anthony

"Remember, no one can make you feel inferior without your consent."

—Eleanor Roosevelt

"Tell us what it is to be a woman so that we may know what it is to be a man."

—Toni Morrison, Nobel Lecture, 1993

Is schizophrenia different in women?

Should patients who are pregnant take medication for schizophrenia?

What is the risk of a postpartum relapse?

More . . .

85. Is schizophrenia different in women?

For many years in the United States and elsewhere, women were placed in psychiatric hospitals for long periods of time and institutionalized simply for having a domineering husband who wanted to "discard her" or coming from a dysfunctional family life. Husbands who wished to rid themselves of their wives could sign commitment papers and claim psychiatric symptoms in their wives in order to do so. Geller and Harris (1994) have documented the histories of typical women of this sort from as early as 1840 through 1945. More humane treatment and legislation against involuntary hospitalization for less than acutely dangerous conditions have abolished these inequities, but they remain documented in the history of psychiatry.

In fact, there is no reason to keep many women hospitalized for long periods of time, as schizophrenia has a much better outcome in women than men overall. Women have a later age of onset than men on average and may also have a different cluster of symptoms and are more likely to have a brief psychotic episode that resolves more quickly than in men. Women also are less aggressive than men and are not prone to committing violent acts as frequently when unmedicated, and thus are not usually a danger to other people. The poorer social outcome for men than women often can be attributed to having a less advanced level of social development by the time of onset than women. Thus, age at onset of the biology of schizophrenia may be the key variable.

Late-onset schizophrenia (over the age of 40) occurs almost exclusively in women. Women are more often diagnosed with schizoaffective disorder and less frequently with paranoid schizophrenia than men, but how much of this difference might be cultural, at least in part, is unknown. Pharmacotherapy in women should also be different because the response of women to medications may differ from men. They require lower doses in order to suppress symptoms, and some serious side effects are more often seen in women than men. Drug trials, however, that specifically compare women with men and that control for various factors that could affect drug levels and thus treatment response (such as cigarette smoking), are far too few. Women tend to be ignored and even eliminated from research clinical trials. The lack of this research is unwarranted, but even to date, some studies do not include women, the reasoning being that hormonal cycles are thought to make interpretation of any study results on women difficult. Thus, unfortunately, recommended treatments and their doses are all based on trials with predominantly male patients.

Hopefully this bias could be changing in the near future. This has been an issue to which the U.S. NIMH is very sensitive. In order for research grants to be funded, the subjects need to be shown to be equally distributed between males and females in accordance with the population frrom which they are drawn.

A common notion to explain sex differences is that **estrogen** levels must have a protective effect on the development of schizophrenia. Some studies show a modulation of the dopamine D-2 receptors by estrogen, and also that estrogen has a weak neuroleptic-like effect. This is not the only explanation for sex differences, however. In fact, genetics also clearly plays a role in actual age of onset. Despite the age of onset for schizophrenia being on average a couple of years later in women than men, when more than one individual within a family has

Estrogen

A female hormone that is produced in the female organs (ovaries). It is produced in different amounts throughout the menstrual cycle and is reduced after menopause in women.

schizophrenia, the age of onset tends to be highly similar regardless of the sex of the affected individuals. This implies that inheritance also influences the age of onset. If the sex differences in schizophrenia are genetic, then a gene that modifies the illness expression, and causes the sex differences noted, may be on the sex chromosomes (DeLisi and Crow, 1989). Although this had been a theory of interest to this writer, it has not received much attention in the current world of large Genome-Wide Genetic Association studies (GWAS). Some of them, in fact, do not examine sex chromosome genes.

86. Should patients who are pregnant take medication for schizophrenia?

Women who take antipsychotic medication, because of its hyperprolactin effects, are less fertile than women who are not on these medications. Exposing the developing infant prenatally or through lactation to antipsychotic medication could also have long-term consequences. The conventional neuroleptics do have an increased risk of congenital malformations, particularly during the earlier weeks of pregnancy (weeks 4 through 10), and we have little data on the newer atypical medications. The establishment of recommended dosing for women during pregnancy has not been adequately studied, nor has any treatment trial been performed comparing different neuroleptic treatments for their subsequent effect on the developing fetus. It also may be that the hormonal modification of the action of some neuroleptics may allow for lower doses to be given during pregnancy, but this needs to be carefully examined. The pharmacologic management of women in the perinatal period when hormonal status suddenly changes is also very important, and little has been described about this condition in the literature.

Having schizophrenia also leads to an increased risk for obstetrical complications, including preterm deliveries and a low-birth-weight infant. The interaction of obstetric complications with use of neuroleptic medications and psychiatric stability is unknown. In general, women with schizophrenia also tend to receive poorer **prenatal** medical care, and this too may lead to complications as a consequence. It is clear that not enough research has been done on pregnancy in schizophrenia. Overall, the risk of withholding medication to suppress psychosis must be weighed against the risk to the fetus and to the mother.

Prenatal

The period between conception and birth.

In addition, women with schizophrenia have higher rates of forced sex and unwanted pregnancies. They may also have a reduced capacity to provide mothering and to respond to their child's needs and thus require special guidance to overcome and deal with these circumstances and deficits.

87. What is the risk of a postpartum relapse?

Special support after birth for women with schizophrenia needs to be intensive, and postpartum relapse prevented or detected early so that treatment can quickly be augmented. The risk of a postpartum psychiatric disorder is higher in women with a prior psychiatric history than those without it, particularly depression and psychosis. The change in hormone levels during the perinatal period may also warrant change in neuroleptic dose. Unfortunately, there have been too many highly publicized cases in the United States of mothers who either have a postpartum relapse of their illness or have a first episode of a psychosis during the postpartum period as long as six months after giving birth. At the extreme, these women can be very harmful to their children and have been known to kill them because of various delusional beliefs, such as in the famous Andrea Yates case. Mrs. Yates had multiple delusions about her children being cursed by the devil, and she acted upon her need to supposedly "end their suffering" by drowning them one by one. Her husband was unaware that she had psychiatric problems and did not pick up on any warning signs. Such tragic events could be avoided with careful recognition and treatment of high-risk postpartum women by healthcare professionals and the education of close family members.

88. Should mothers with schizophrenia breast-feed infants?

Postpartum lactation and breast-feeding may augment the higher prolactin levels already present during conventional antipsychotic treatment. Breast milk, however, likely excretes neuroleptics, and thus breast-feeding should be cautioned against in medicated patients. We do not know the effect of neuroleptics on the developing infant but assume that there could be lasting effects on the brain and nervous system. There are no studies of children of breast-feeding patients on neuroleptics, nor are there studies of the new atypical neuroleptics to see whether they are safer than old generation neuroleptics for women. It is presently unknown whether any of these medications, including antidepressants, affect brain growth and development, although it is now known that the SSRI antidepressants can increase brain-derived neurotrophic factor (BDNF) and thus must have some effect, beneficial or not, on the developing brain. Nevertheless, it is recommended that women on these medications do not breast-feed their children.

It is hoped that the pharmaceutical industry will take the responsibility to investigate these important issues in the near future.

89. Can estrogen for birth control help suppress symptoms?

Often, women who have schizophrenia and are sexually active do not use contraceptives and frequently are not compliant with oral contraceptives; thus, if warranted, the use of long-acting contraceptive medications is the method of choice. Whether these treatments augment the effects of antipsychotic medication has been little studied. Although there have been some reports to suggest this, as mentioned previously here, large-scale studies of women have not been a focus in research. It is also of interest that drug trials of the new antipsychotics that do include women do not standardize whether women are administered oral contraceptives. Again, systematic trials need to be supported by the pharmaceutical companies, because a few small studies suggest an augmenting antipsychotic effect of estrogen in women.

90. Can schizophrenia be exacerbated during and after menopause?

When a change occurs in hormone levels, symptoms may re-emerge, and such is the case in the perimenopausal years. There is much literature to suggest that estrogen is neuroprotective, and thus with lowering of its levels, the brain is more vulnerable. If a patient is taking neuroleptics, the dose may need to be raised. In addition, there is some indication that taking an estrogen receptor modulator, such as raloxifene, may be helpful for both the specific disease symptoms and also cognition. Most important, a patient with schizophrenia taking antipsychotic medication is particularly at risk for low bone density and osteoporosis as well as cardiac and other physiological disorders, and should be monitored closely.

PART 10

The Homeless and Schizophrenia

"There was a table set out under the tree... and the March Hare and the Hatter were having tea at it: a Dormouse was sitting between them, fast asleep, and the other two were using it as a cushion, resting their elbows on it, and talking over its head. 'Very uncomfortable for the Dormouse,' thought Alice, 'only, as it's asleep, I suppose it doesn't mind.'"

—Lewis Carroll, *Alice in Wonderland*

How prevalent is schizophrenia among the homeless?

What causes homelessness, and what is being done to prevent it?

More...

91. How prevalent is schizophrenia among the homeless?

Many of us walk and jump over homeless men and woman dressed in multiple layers of old clothes sleeping on city sidewalks or heated grates, possibly not understanding how they could feel and rationalizing that their sleeping souls are oblivious to the cold and pain. The argument given by some is that the homeless prefer living that way, and if given housing would choose not to take it. Do we know, however, whether those that are homeless have the capacity to make this decision? Recent research surveys indicate that many of the urban homeless would be diagnosed with schizophrenia. Perhaps because of their illness, they are too disorganized and incapable of seeking shelter or finding permanent independent housing.

Historically, before the rise of public mental institutions run by the states, it was widely known that a large number of homeless individuals lined urban streets, a high percentage of whom had mental illness. It was, in fact, in part for this very reason that psychiatric institutions came into existence in large numbers (detailed in Torrey, 1989). The community mental health center concept that was promoted in the 1960s, combined with the wide-scale use of neuroleptic medications in public psychiatric hospitals, produced a movement for reintegrating these institutionalized people with schizophrenia back into the community. This program, funded by the federal government in the United States and similar such projects in other countries, established outpatient mental health centers within local communities. These local centers largely failed, however. Primarily, there were not enough community care homes with adequate facilities for patients to be moved to, and the funds provided were inadequate to keep the centers and the corresponding residential facilities maintained. Thus, this so-called worldwide deinstitutionalization came full-circle again to massive increases in homelessness.

Another problem was the lack of coordination of the inpatient care with referral systems to the community mental health centers. Thus, the centers treated many more mildly ill patients who were not in need of hospitalization, whereas those who were released from the psychiatric hospitals had difficulty becoming integrated into the healthcare system. These newly released patients would then not continue their medication and lose the ability to care for themselves and plan daily living and coping strategies, and so they took to the streets.

Regardless of psychiatric status, people living at or below the federal poverty level are the most vulnerable to experiencing a homeless episode. The estimated annual projections account for 6.3% to 9.6% of the total U.S. population in poverty and 6.2% to 9.3% of children in poverty. Among homeless women, the prevalence of psychiatric disorders in one study was 71%, with substance abuse the leading disorder (43%), followed by anxiety disorders (35%) and then schizophrenia (12%). Many other studies find similar rates for schizophrenia among the homeless (both men and women) ranging from 2% to 45% internationally and with an average of 11% worldwide, with rates somewhat higher in women than men and higher in the young and the chronically homeless. Suicide rates are also higher in the homeless in general than non-homeless, regardless of psychiatric diagnosis.

Another report, *Homelessness: Programs and the People They Serve*, is a set of publications and a collaborative effort of the Census Bureau and the U.S. Department of Housing and Urban Development. The study's findings are eye-opening at the very least: 38% report evidence of alcohol use problems in the past month; 26% report drug use problems; 39% report some evidence of mental health problems; and 66% report indicators of one or more of these problems. (See the Appendix for details about where to find more information about homelessness.)

92. What causes homelessness, and what is being done to prevent it?

On a general level, homelessness is caused by poverty and unemployment, but how a person gets to that extreme level and transitions to living on a street is more complex. Estimates show that worldwide at least 1.3 million people are homeless, that is, without even basic minimal shelter. Even in a booming economy, at least 2.3 million adults and children, or nearly 1% of the U.S. population, are likely to experience a spell of homelessness at least once during a year. In 2009, reflecting an economic recession world-wide, the statistics were even higher with higher unemployment rates and a failed credit market for homes. In 2014, at the last estimate, the National Alliance to End Homelessness estimates that on any given night 500,000–600,000 people are homeless (www.endhomelessness.org).

Fleeing from violence is a predominant reason for women to be homeless, which differs markedly from male homelessness. Homelessness in people with schizophrenia has been blamed on a failure of the mental health system to provide adequate care for patients after they are discharged from the hospital as stated above. There continues to exist, however, the possibility that the nature of schizophrenia itself and its negative symptoms create homelessness, not for economic reasons, but because these people fail to use cognitive planning abilities to provide themselves with proper shelter, a very basic aspect of human survival.

New York City is an interesting example of how homelessness was seemingly decreased over a short period of time. Over two decades ago, there were many more homeless people on the streets of New York than there are now. What reduced this number so drastically? It was not the better treatment of patients with schizophrenia or the "war on street drug abuse" taking an effect, but it was rather the authority of then-mayor of New York, Rudy Giuliani. His goal was to move all of the homeless off the streets and from public parks, building shelters, but mainly using police force to take them off the streets and off of park benches at night, placing them mostly in jails when they did not go to shelters. If a homeless person is not acutely harmful to himself or others, he or she cannot be forced into psychiatric treatment and medication. He or she can, however, be picked up for "loitering" or other crimes and be placed in jail. Often, mentally ill persons confined to jail unfortunately do not receive proper medical treatment.

Other cities and private charities have established large public shelters for the homeless that are particularly important during the cold months of the year. These shelters, if organized well, have social workers who facilitate placing the homeless in housing with governmental supplemental funds, and people who facilitate the homeless receiving the medical and psychiatric treatment they need. However, the shelters can also be tough places, particularly for women, who report rapes and abuse; both men and woman may find that their meager possessions or money are stolen at night when they sleep, and street drugs are all too prevalent around the shelters. Most shelters also require that those who inhabit them are not inside during the daytime hours, and thus they sit in the libraries or other public buildings waiting for the night to come when the weather is cold, and in the parks during the warmer months. Other homeless individuals, who have the mental capacity to do so, can be found migrating from city to city, i.e., the warmer climates in winter months, and colder cities in the summer. These individuals, unfortunately, are not in any one place long enough to acquire consistent health care or social aid.

Homelessness remains one of America's most complicated and important social issues. Chronic poverty, coupled with physical, mental, and other disabilities, have combined with rapid changes in society, the workplace, and local housing markets to make many people vulnerable to becoming homeless. With the enactment of the Stewart B. McKinney Homeless Assistance Act of 1987, Congress recognized the need to supplement "mainstream" federally funded housing and human services programs with funding that was specifically targeted to assist homeless people. The program that was established includes provisions for emergency shelters, transitional housing programs, permanent housing programs for formerly homeless people, programs distributing vouchers for emergency accommodation, programs accepting vouchers in exchange for giving emergency accommodation, food pantries, soup kitchens, mobile food programs, physical healthcare programs, mental healthcare programs, alcohol/drug programs, HIV/AIDS programs, outreach programs, drop-in centers, and migrant camps that provide emergency shelter for homeless people that seek temporary farming jobs from one state to another (the so-called "migrant workers").

Thus, over the past couple of decades, there has been tremendous growth in services for the homeless. The shelter and housing capacity in the United States within the homeless assistance network grew by 220% between 1988 and 1996, from 275,000 beds to almost 608,000 beds in 1996. Growth slowed in the subsequent decades, however, and the economic crisis of 2008 as well as political inertia meant that as of 2013, the total number of available spaces (including shelter beds, transitional housing, and permanent supportive housing) was about 708,000 beds. Soup kitchen and meal distribution services in central cities nearly quadrupled between 1987 and 1996, from 97,000 to 382,100 meals on an average day in winter 1996. Nationally, these programs expected to serve almost 570,000 meals, approximately one-third of which were served outside of central cities. The U.S. Department of Agriculture (USDA) statistics on food insecurity, however, noted an even sharper increase in food insecurity among poor households in the mid-2000s. Some food banks reported increases in use of as much as 50% between the 2007 financial crisis and 2014. Other types of homeless services have also increased, including health services, outreach programs, and drop-in centers—yet simultaneously, many cities are still aggressively promoting and enforcing laws that criminalize homelessness and authorizing police to confiscate the possessions of homeless people, remove them from city parks or other public areas, and in some cases arrest them. For homeless individuals with schizophrenia, especially those with paranoid tendencies, these practices may exacerbate existing mental health issues and put them at even greater risk. (*Source*: https://www.hudexchange.info/resources/documents/ahar-2013-part1.pdf)

PART 11

Legal and Ethical Issues

"They have said that he was like George Washington and his only crime was his unswerving and uncompromising patriotism, that he was not guilty of treason, that he was not a Fascist, that he was not anti-Semitic, that he was deprived of his rights to a fair trial, and that he was held as a political prisoner. The biggest myth, however, was that he was insane."

—E. Fuller Torrey (1984) on beginning his book about Ezra Pound's psychiatric hospitalization

"The Hadamar gas chamber was set up in the basement...At the conclusion of the admission procedures the nurse would tell the patients they were to have a nice shower...The unsuspecting patients would have no objection to such a suggestion...and the director of the Hadamar center presided over a cocktail party commemorating the killing of their ten-thousandth patient."

—Hugh Gregory Gallagher, *By Trust Betrayed*, 1995

What does "involuntary" hospital commitment involve?

What is the legal insanity defense?

Do patients with schizophrenia have the capacity to give informed consent for research and medical procedures?

More...

93. What does "involuntary" hospital commitment involve?

Many years ago, a disgruntled husband could put away his wife for years in a psychiatric hospital. Now, however, there are laws to prevent this. Although the rules of each state and each country vary, in general, when a person is acutely ill and unable to have the capacity to understand what is happening in order to make personal decisions and he or she is considered a danger to himself or others, he or she can be held involuntarily in psychiatric hospitalized treatment for a short period of time, renewable by two physicians. Court hearings can also resolve this if the patients continue to request hospital discharge, but the doctors feel otherwise.

Sometimes outpatient commitment is also made mandatory so that patients are required to continue medication even when they do not have insight into the fact that they are ill and in need of the long-term medications. In this case, the only way they would be allowed by law to stay out of the hospital and in the community is if they comply with the court-ordered medication. Sometimes the law can be on the side of the patient who might still be harmful and manage to conceal this behavior. If patients seem rational and fail to admit their intentions, there is no way of keeping them in the hospital confined against their will, as was the case with the patient from Long Island who was able to conceal his pathological wish to kill his wife from doctors and nursing staff and left the grounds of Pilgrim State Hospital on a day pass, only to murder his wife shortly afterward.

A related issue is whether a psychiatrist has the responsibility to divulge information received during the doctor–patient relationship if it could imply harm toward another person. This controversy has recently surfaced in the international news, as discussions have persisted about a pilot of a Lufthansa-owned airline putatively having crashed it into a mountain, killing all individuals aboard. Investigations revealed that the pilot had been in psychiatric treatment. Although details have not been revealed about the case, if he had been in treatment with a psychiatrist, would that psychiatrist have the duty to break confidentiality and warn appropriate officials should danger be suspected. The laws for such are different in each country and in the case of some, psychiatrists could be more at risk for losing the ability to practice should confidentiality be broken than if not. One legal case that changed laws in the U.S., known as the Tarasoff Case, arose in California in the mid 1970s. A patient let his therapist know that he felt like harming a female friend who had rebuffed him because she did not want an intimate relationship with him. Although the therapist called the police to pick up the patient, having diagnosed him with paranoid schizophrenia and considering him to be dangerous, he failed to warn the intended victim, who was indeed eventually murdered by the patient. This case was quite controversial and went from local courts to the California Supreme Court in two separate parts. The court rulings made it the responsibility of a doctor and/or any therapist not only to care for the patient, but to warn an intended victim about possible harm. The police, who had spoken to the patient and ultimately set him free, were exonerated, and the responsibility was placed entirely on the clinician. In another case in North Carolina, a psychiatrist was held responsible for a former patient's murderous spree 8 months after he was no longer in the psychiatrist's care. A jury found the psychiatrist culpable because when he last saw the patient, the doctor did not follow through to make sure his recommendations for seeking further care and continuing medications were adhered to.

Nevertheless, patients who have been hospitalized in state or other public hospital locked wards are often there for months. Most have not committed the kind of crimes mentioned earlier, but are confined inside and it often feels like jail. As they become stable, the ward staff must then decide whether they are capable of having privileges to be free to walk on the grounds of the hospital or even go on passes into the nearby town. These are often difficult decisions and care is taken when making them weighing the patient's ability to conduct his/herself responsibility and not be harmful to himself or others.

94. What is the legal insanity defense?

An insanity defense is a legal term that excuses people with mental illness from legal responsibility for their crime. Many jurisdictions even allow insanity defenses to be entered on behalf of an offender even when the defendant objects. By far the most frequent psychiatric condition associated with an insanity defense is schizophrenia. In forming professional opinions about a particular case, psychiatrists may need to change their views depending on the actual *legal* definition of insanity, which may differ from one jurisdiction to the next. Psychiatrists are not accustomed to using this term in the sense meant by the law. Someone can be acutely psychotic but still able to understand the difference between right and wrong actions. Someone may commit a criminal act without understanding his or her actions (e.g., the man who kills his grandparents because "voices" told him to do it and because he "knew" that they were about to kill him, or the woman who drove her children into a lake to drown them because she "knew" they were devils). Did he or she know that they were doing something wrong? Did the man commit a crime who drove his car through the White House gates because he thought that it was the only way to let the president know his opinions?

In March, 1981, in Washington, DC, John Hinckley, Jr. shot both president Reagan and James Brady. He was found not guilty by reason of insanity and sent to St Elizabeths Hospital. Although he is on medication, he is also now quietly living in a community setting and his discharge is being considered because psychiatrists believe he is no longer a danger to society. However, his discharge to live in the community or with his mother will be made very difficult because of the publicity associated with his case and the nature of his previous delusions and how he acted upon them in relation to national political interests. In addition, since his trial, the laws for the insanity defense have tightened. Many states would like to eliminate the insanity defense entirely because medication may not cure some criminal behavior. After having murdered once, a person may not hesitate to do it again.

In New York in 1980, an Insanity Defense Reform Act was passed even before the publicity of the Hinckley trial, and specified the procedures necessary for releasing persons to the community who were found not guilty of a criminal offense by reason of insanity. The most important condition was participation in an outpatient treatment program. Some follow-up studies, however, have found that one-fourth to one-third of these patients were rearrested, many for crimes of violence, and others were rehospitalized and their releases revoked. These people obviously constitute a special group of patients that on hospital release need long-term treatment and social guidance in the community with close follow-up.

At the more recent trial to decide whether the man who opened fire in an Aurora, Colorado movie theatre, killing several people, the defense, pleading "not guilty by reason of insanity," brought in a renowned psychiatrist whose expertise was schizophrenia. She stated to the court that there was no doubt in her mind that the defendant committed the crime because he was delusional and he would not have committed the crime if he did not have the described delusions. It is not clear where that statement leads, however, as he still could have understood what was morally right and what was wrong. Thus, the jury concluded that he was guilty and did not agree with the insanity plea.

In some countries, such as in Cuba during the 1970s, and Ireland in the 1800s, as well as other parts of the United Kingdom, the criminally insane were released but were deported to other countries. Although this obviously does not solve the problem for the patients, the country of origin felt collectively safer. Interestingly, some surveys actually show that those with psychotic diagnoses, such as schizophrenia, tend to be most of the criminals who obtain insanity defenses, whereas those with a prior criminal history, personality disorders, or drug and alcohol charges tend not to enter an insanity plea. Despite this, there is still a racial disparity so that whites are more likely to be successful with an insanity defense than people from minority backgrounds in the United States. Some thought should be given to such biases.

Another issue is whether someone found mentally ill can be executed for a crime in states that have the death penalty. Some state courts have ruled that criminals could not be forcibly medicated in order to make them competent for execution.

There have on the other side been historical political abuses of psychiatric diagnoses and the insanity plea. During the late 1970s, the World Psychiatric Association was investigating Russian psychiatrists for the hospitalization of political dissidents under the guise of having a particular form of politically invented schizophrenia. More recently, the same practices have been suggested to be taking place in China. Some people have suggested that when Ezra Pound, the poet, was hospitalized at St. Elizabeth's in Washington, DC for many years, it was because of his extreme anti-American political views—not because he was psychotic. The 2009 movie *Changeling,* nominated for an Academy Award in the movie industry, depicts the corrupt practice in the 1920s of hospitalizing people who did not comply with Los Angeles police actions on psychiatric inpatient units; thus, a young mother who had lost her child and pestered the police to continue to search for him, was placed on a psychiatric ward, told she was delusional, and given ECT.

Patient who abuse the system certainly exist as well. Someone who commits a crime can also be astute enough to know that an insanity defense might mean confinement in a psychiatric hospital until the psychiatric condition "resolves" to allow them to regain their freedom. Thus, symptoms can be mimicked for a time, and the criminal then feigns that they are resolved. The dilemma is that the only way one can diagnose schizophrenia is by the patient's admission of symptoms and observation of his or her behavior. Sometimes a distinction between malingering and the real illness cannot be ascertained; other times, by interviewing a relative or close friend who has observed the patient over time and at other occasions, a more comprehensive picture of the person emerges.

The other side to this issue is that people with mental illness are often placed in prison instead of a psychiatric hospital and often do not receive the treatment that they need for their illness. Often they have no insight into their illness, and they deny symptoms when prodded. It is only the astute psychiatrist who can tell these two opposite conditions apart.

The following is an example of the currently existing problems in prisons when it comes to the management of people with serious mental illness (published in *The New York Times*, February 28, 2005):

> "In City's Jails, Missed Signals Open Way to Season of Suicides" by Paul von Zielbauer "Prison Health Services Cares for More Than 100,000 Inmates Each Year at Nine Riker's Island Prison in New York City and a 10th Jail in Manhattan"...Mistakes and Missteps in a Season of Suicides" *Prison Health Services and New York City's correction system share the blame for a spate of inmate suicides in 2003, government investigators said....* The New York Times' *year-long examination of Prison Health Services, the biggest commercial provider of medical care to inmates, found instances of disturbing deaths and other troubling treatment. The warnings were right there in her medical file: a childhood of sexual abuse, a diagnosis of manic depression, a suicide attempt at age 13—all noted when Carina Montes arrived at Riker's Island in September 2002. State investigators said that none of them were ever seen by the mental health specialist caring for her. He could never track down the file,*

> *which by December included another troubling fact: Ms. Montes had been placed on suicide watch by a jail social worker. Not that the suicide watch was terribly reliable; it depended in part on inmates paid 39 cents an hour to check on their suicidal peers. In her 5 months at Riker's, investigators later discovered that Ms. Montes never saw a psychiatrist.*

It did not, however, take a psychiatrist to pick up on the alarms she sounded near the end, when another inmate saw her tearing bed sheets and threatening to kill herself. But the guard who was called had no idea she was on suicide watch, did not notice the sheets and never reported the incident. Six hours later, Ms. Montes was dead, hanging from a sheet tied to a ventilation grate. She was 29. Her offense: shoplifting 30 lipsticks. The death of Carina Montes was one in a spate of suicides in New York City jails in 2003—six in just 6 months, more than in any similar stretch since 1985. None of these people had been convicted of the charges that put them in jail. But in Ms. Montes's death and four of the five others, government investigators reached a stinging judgment about one or both of the authorities responsible for their safety: Prison Health Services, the nation's largest for-profit provider of inmate medical care, and the city correction system. In their reports, investigators faulted a system in which patients' charts were missing, alerts about despondent inmates were lost or unheeded, and neither medical personnel nor correction officers were properly trained in preventing suicide, the leading cause of deaths in American jails. As this book goes to print, a young woman written about in the newspaper was found having committed suicide in a jail cell. Her crime was having been picked up by police for a traffic violation and she was held overnight in jail until she could appear in court.

95. Why participate in research, and can patients with schizophrenia have the capacity to give informed consent for research and medical procedures?

Many of the major academic institutions have psychiatrists who conduct research on schizophrenia. Currently, relatively little is known about this disease compared with most other medical disorders; thus, research of multiple kinds needs to continue, with adequate funding from public sources. Although many theories about schizophrenia exist, the fact still is that there is no biological test for it, there are no symptoms that are specific to schizophrenia, and there is no preventive measure one can take to avoid getting this illness. We only know that it has an inherited component of some sort and that it appears usually in early adulthood or late adolescence, that it has some sex differences, and that medications can suppress the symptoms, such as having delusionary perceptions and auditory hallucinations, as long as these medications are taken continuously as prescribed.

Research is desperately needed to find drugs that target the cause of illness and to find treatments that prevent the chronic course before it begins. It is also needed to find measures to improve the quality of life in those people who do develop a chronic illness and are only marginally able to live out their lives outside of an institution. Participating in research studies generally does not help the individual directly but can, in the future, benefit others who develop the illness. Often, however, being in a research study means that better care is available to oneself and one's family because the researchers are generally well recognized as experts in their field and will know where and how to obtain the best treatment, although this is not always the case. Access to care is then facilitated, and earlier detection may result for other family members that can lead then to a better outcome.

NIMH often lists various research studies on their website. Researchers advertise through clinics, hospitals, and support groups such as NAMI, so that if you would like to be a part of some of these studies that are generally not risky, this should be possible. In addition, the rights of individuals who participate in research are protected by an oversight Institutional Review Board (IRB). IRBs approve written research protocols and stress that the subject must be competent to provide written informed consent, that is they must understand the risks and benefits of the research procedures before participating and understand that it is voluntary and thus he/she may withdraw without having his/her clinical treatment with the most established treatments affected. Many years ago, research had the potential to be abusive because there were no laws to govern how it could be done. These practices have changed considerably over the past couple of decades, and human subjects protection in research is now a very sensitive issue internationally.

Stabilized chronic patients with schizophrenia who are currently functioning outside of a hospital in a group home or independently almost always have the capacity to understand the information that is being presented. The question has remained about those who are incapable of living outside of the hospital, who are in a supervised environment, or who are experiencing an acute psychotic episode. In general, people with schizophrenia still have the capacity to understand instructions if things are explained clearly and slowly, and they are given the opportunity to ask questions. They also have decisional capacity and the ability to exercise their will voluntarily if the time is taken to explain information. Their attention span and preoccupation with their thought disorders and hallucinations during an acute episode makes them appear not to understand. To obtain such evidence of capacity, patients can be explained things carefully and then asked questions to see whether they understood. Also, structured capacity tests can be given to each patient. There is great sensitivity now among legislators, academics, researchers, and institutional review boards for human research, and careful rules must be followed to obtain written informed consent from subjects for all kinds of research studies. People who have diseases that reduce their capacity to understand what they are participating in, depending on the nature of a study, or procedure can have legal guardians give consent for them. They may also need a legal guardian to take care of their every day affairs, particularly finances.

With respect to research participation, progress aimed toward finding better treatments for these disorders is essential; thus, alternative provisions, such as the ability to have a legal guardian to consent who can weigh the risks and benefits carefully, are important. Unfortunately, our country, as well as others, has in its too recent history evidence of abuses by researchers of groups of people who cannot protect their individual rights, such as those who are mentally retarded or demented or those who are prisoners. Thus, legislation has been enacted to safeguard these people from being subject to forceful participation in research.

PART 12

Living with Schizophrenia and Recovery

"Whatever meaning people feel can be derived from their personal suffering, to live without pain would, I believe, be even more meaningful, even more human."

—Excerpt from *Unconditional Life: Mastering the Forces that Shape Personal Reality* by Deepak Chopra*

Can people with schizophrenia recover?

What are the origins of the stigma attached to having schizophrenia?

Can a person with schizophrenia be professionally creative?

More...

96. Can people with schizophrenia recover?

Until recently, schizophrenia was thought of as an illness from which one would not recover. However, a large proportion of patients (larger than thought in the past), appear to do quite well after an initial bout with illness. Outcome has certainly improved with the use of medications early one in the illness course and with the earlier recognition of signs and symptoms of the illness before they progress to hospitalization.

The word "recovery" means different things to different people. Recovery itself has been recognized as a whole process and way of thinking about one's goals. It could mean no longer needing medication and becoming the person one was prior to becoming ill, or it could also mean perhaps having different goals, but living independently and feeling satisfied with one's life and interpersonal relationships. One can still feel recovered while continuing to take medications daily as well. How long one needs to take medication is an open question that has not adequately been answered. Over time, the longer one goes without symptoms of schizophrenia in years, the more likely it is that the medication can be reduced and a trial without it implemented. However, this should be done under the close supervision of a psychiatrist who may easily recognize early signs of relapse. There is no set protocol that has yet come from clinical trials to determine how long a period of recovery must be before removing medication. This will likely vary from person to person.

97. What are the origins of the stigma attached to having schizophrenia?

The word *stigma* dates back to the ancient Greeks, who defined this as something unusual about someone's body that suggests something bad and immoral. This term is widely used to be synonymous with something disgraceful or of which to be ashamed. In general, something that is *stigmatized* is a trait that turns people away from the individual who has it, as it is assumed that this person is less than human. Anyone who does not behave within the norms accepted by society is stigmatized in a similar manner to minority racial stigmatization. For many decades, families who had affected psychotic individuals would hide them in attics, closets, and basements; this was more easily done in rural than urban settings. There was the fear of a family being stigmatized if one of its members had a mental illness. Until recently, having depression was similar. Over the last decade, however, when individuals who are well respected in the community have gone public with their illnesses (such as Kay Jamison, Mike Wallace, Margot Kidder, Brian Wilson, and others) and published books on the topic, awareness that depression and bipolar disorder are diseases that can be treated has slowly taken place. People with these illnesses may still be stigmatized, but less so than in the past. Public education and awareness have helped to reduce the stigma. It has been less so for schizophrenia, probably because people with this illness do not make good advocates for themselves.

Their prominent language and thought disorders, along with residual negative symptoms, as well as come cognitive impairment, prevent them from speaking out and becoming proactive. Thus, it has been up to their families to form public advocacy groups. The many support groups having members coming from well-respected families in the community have helped to establish public networks for regular meetings and education and to lobby for the rights of the disabled mentally ill. With new medications and the return of people with schizophrenia to productive lives and with the knowledge that these are not people to be feared, stigma can be reduced.

98. Can a person with schizophrenia be professionally creative?

Many famous examples of creative people with schizophrenia are available, such as John Nash who received the Nobel Prize for his work on game theory, the artist Van Gogh, or several musicians. Creativity is usually more frequently associated with manic-depressive psychosis than schizophrenia because in mania there is a flurry of grandiose thoughts and an excess of energy, whereas in schizophrenia, there is withdrawal and a loss of internal drive as well as disorganization of thoughts. The latter do not lend themselves to creative products. It is usually the exceptional person (such as John Nash) who was highly creative prior to having full-blown schizophrenia and who, although never returning to that fully creative intellectually productive state again, is still able to retain some semblance of that level of functioning even after the chronic illness sets in. John Nash is famous for what he accomplished at a young age before the onset of his psychosis; he was never as productive as he would have been had he not developed schizophrenia, although he remained for many years on the Princeton campus able to inspire students to be productive in the field of mathematics.

99. Should a person with schizophrenia drive a car?

Losing one's driver's license or having to forfeit the ability to drive is a loss of independence that is very difficult for anyone to adjust to, and not any less so for people with schizophrenia. However, for the safety of others on the road, it may be that on an individual basis, particularly for a patient who is either unreliably taking their medications or whose symptoms never fully abate, that others will have to firmly remove his/her permission to drive. For example, I had a patient who entered the hospital after the last of a series of car accidents, having run a red light because he became unusually frightened seeing a police car in his rear-view window when he stopped at an intersection. His baseline paranoia had gotten the best of him and he rammed into another car; luckily, no one was injured. Yet his family did not want to take the steps of having his license removed. I was the person who had to inform authorities that this person should not be able to have the privilege of being on the road.

"Road rage" has become a problem on some city highways, particularly when traffic is heavy and people do not have the patience to wait their turn or deal with the driver next to them who is not keeping up with traffic. If someone has a mental illness, particularly with paranoid and irritable traits, it may be difficult to deal with such other drivers, either because paranoia toward them can manifest or because the stress of the drive can not be dealt with. Thus, this also must be taken into account when considering the readiness for driving of someone recovering from a schizophrenia episode.

As reaction-time tests and simulated driving studies have shown, people with schizophrenia tend not to be able to respond as quickly in a coordinated manner to unexpected changes in driving conditions. Although there are no known statistics on the rates of accidents in people with schizophrenia, you would expect that it could be significantly higher for people with schizophrenia than in the general population.

Nevertheless, some statistics show that 50% of outpatients with schizophrenia drive automobiles. Antipsychotic medication can affect the ability to drive, although some indication exists that atypical antipsychotics may not have this effect. However, providing that a person is not on a sedating medication that causes drowsiness and thus affects driving response, patients with schizophrenia who have been stabilized and are not preoccupied with unsuppressed symptoms are likely responsible drivers on roads that are uncomplicated, short distances, and generally not normally stressful driving stretches. Under no circumstances should a patient drive when he or she is experiencing an acute episode that is not stabilized with medication. Whether a patient should drive an automobile should be considered on an individual basis. In the future, state driving tests may be modified so that all individuals might be required to take a stimulus-response test. Certainly other medical conditions, such as substance abuse, aging, and other neurological diseases, can hamper driving ability, as well as the newer problem of addiction to cell phones and text messaging while driving in otherwise normal individuals. Schizophrenia should not be singled out.

100. What support groups, books, and websites can I go to for help?

A list of support groups, websites, and books can be found under Resources. This book has been about public awareness of schizophrenia and is written so that the misperceptions about this illness based only on scientific half-truths will not occur. Schizophrenia is on the extreme edge of the wide range of what the world calls "normality"; however, that is defined in each culture and at each point in time. It is an illness, however, by virtue of the pain and destruction it causes to those afflicted. With the eventual development of future medications that target its biology, this illness has the hope of being prevented. No one should feel shame or be stigmatized because he or she suffers from schizophrenia; rather, he or she should receive the best treatment from those who are trained to give it and then live their lives to their best potential.

Resources

Support Groups

The most extensive and prominent support group in the United States is the National Alliance on Mental Illness (NAMI), which has local chapters throughout the country. The national office is located at 3803 North Fairfax Drive, Suite 100, Arlington, Virginia 22203; telephone: 1-703-524-7600; E-mail: info@NAMI.org; Helpline: 800-950-6264; website: *www.NAMI.org*.

Each state and major city has local chapters that can also be found through the national website or by independently Googling them.

In Canada, the largest national support group is the Canadian Alliance on Mental Illness and Mental Health (CAMIMH); 141 Laurier Avenue West, Suite 702, Ottawa, ON KIP 5J3; Telephone: 613-237-2144, ext 323; Website: *www.camimh.ca*; Children's Helpline: 1-800-668-6868. Adults are referred to the Canadian Mental Health Association at 1110-151 Slater Street, Ottawa, ON KIP 5H3; website: *www.cmha.ca*

In addition, Canada has the Schizophrenia Society of Canada: 100-4 Fort Street, Winnipeg, MB R3C1C4, Canada; Phone: 204-786-1616; E-mail: info@schizophrenia.ca; Website: *www.schizophrenia.ca*

In the United Kingdom, the best support group is Schizophrenia, a National Emergency (SANE), which is located at Saint Mark's Studios, 14 Chillingworth Road, Islington, London N78QJ; Telephone: 020-7375-1002; E-mail: info@sane.org.uk; Helpline: 0300-304-7000; website: *www.sane.org.uk*.

In Germany, the German Alliance for Mental Health is quite active throughout Germany; Reinhardtstrasse 14, 10117 Berlin, Germany; Phone: 49(0) 30 240477-214 or 213; E-mail: Koordination@seelischegesundheit.net; website: *www.seelischegesiendheit.net*

Australia has the Mental Illness Fellowship of Australia, Inc; 5 Cooke Tce, Wayville, SA 5034; Telephone: 08-8272-1018; E-mail: MIFA@MIFA.org.au; Website: *www.MIFA.org.au*; Helpline: 1800-985-944

Resources for Cognitive Behavioral Therapy

Cognitive behavioral therapy (CBT) resources referred to in Question 39 include:

The Albert Ellis Institute [formerly the Institute for Rational-Emotive Therapy]
45 East 65th Street, New York, NY 10021
1-800-323-4738
http://www.rebt.org

The Beck Institute
GSB Building, City Line and Belmont Avenues
Suite 700
Bala Cynwyd, PA 19004-1610
1-610-664-3020
http://www.beckinstitute.org

National Association of
Cognitive-Behavioral Therapists
P.O. Box 2195
Weirton, WV 26062
1-800-853-1135
http://www.nacbt.org

Homelessness

Information about homelessness and what is being done about it is available from the U.S. Department of Housing and Urban Development's Office of Policy Development and Research at 1-800-245-2691 (*www.hud.gov/offices/cpd/homeless/*) and at this link and address: National Alliance to End Homelessness, (http://www.endhomelessness.org/), 1518 K Street NW, Suite 206,Washington, DC 20005; 1-202-638-1526; naeh@naeh.org.

Recommended Books

The following books can provide further information about schizophrenia and related disorders and can provide a source of comfort for families, friends, and individuals who have been diagnosed with schizophrenia. A more complete reference list for those books and manuscripts quoted in the text appears below.

Andreasen NC (April 2001). *Brave New Brain: Conquering Mental Illness in the Era of the Genome*. Oxford: Oxford University Press.

Jamison KR (1995). *An Unquiet Mind: A Memoir of Mood and Madness*. New York: Alfred A. Knopf.

Jamison KR (1999). *Night Falls Fast: Understanding Suicide*. New York: Alfred A. Knopf.

Morrison J (2014). *DSM-5 Made Easy*. New York: The Guilford Press.

Mueser KT and Gingerich S (2006). *The Complete Family Guide to Schizophrenia: Helping Your Loved One Get the Most Out of Life*. New York: Guilford Press.

Saks ER (2007). *The Center Cannot Hold: My Journey through Madness*. New York: Hyperion.

Torrey EF (2013). *Surviving Schizophrenia: A Family Manual, 6th ed.* New York: HarperCollins.

Torrey EF (2008). *The Insanity Offense*. New York: WW Norton & Co.

Torrey EF (1997). *Out of the Shadows: Confronting America's Mental Illness Crisis*. New York: John Wiley & Sons.

U.S. Department of Health and Human Services (2012). *Schizophrenia: Causes, Symptoms, Signs, Diagnosis and Treatments*. Washington, DC: USDHHS.

Recommended Websites

National Institute of Mental Health website:
http://www.nimh.nih.gov/health/topics/schizophrenia/index.shtml

If, for some reason, these links does not work, try the NIMH home page at *http://www.nimh.nih.gov/.*

International Mental Health Research Organization (IMHRO): One Mind Institute: Global Innovation for Brain Research Website:
www.IMHRO.org

Brain and Behavior Research Foundation website:
https://bbrfoundation.org

Schizophrenia Research Forum website:
www.schizophreniaforum.org

References

American Psychiatric Association (2013). *Diagnostic and Statistical Manual of Mental Disorders,* 5th ed., Arlington, Virginia: American Psychiatric Association Press.

Andreasen NC (2001). *Brave New Brain: Conquering Mental Illness in the Era of the Genome.* Oxford: Oxford University Press.

Bak M, Myin-Germeys I, Hanssen M, Bijl R, Vollebergh W, Delespaul P, van Os J (2003). When does experience of psychosis result in a need for care? A prospective general population study. *Schizophr Bull* 29(2):349–358.

Chopra D (1991). *Unconditional Life: Discovering the Power to Fulfill Your Dreams.* New York: Bantam Books.

Crow TJ (1990). The continuum of psychosis and its genetic origins. *Br J Psychiatry* 156:788–797.

Crow TJ (1997). Is schizophrenia the price that Homo sapiens pays for language? *Schizophr Res* 28:127–141.

DeLisi LE (ed.) (1990). *Depression in Schizophrenia.* Washington, DC: American Association Press.

DeLisi LE (2000). Unifying the concept of psychosis through brain morphology. In: Maneros A, Angst J (eds.) (2000). *Bipolar Disorders: 100 Years After Manic Depressive Insanity.* The Netherlands: Kluwer.

DeLisi LE (2001). Speech disorder in schizophrenia: Review of the literature and new study of the relation to uniquely human capacity for language. *Schizophr Bull* 27:481–496.

DeLisi LE, Crow TJ (1989). Evidence for an X chromosome locus for schizophrenia. *Schizophr Bull* 15:431–440.

El-Hai J (2004). *The Lobotomist: A Maverick Medical Genius and his Tragic Quest to Rid the World of Mental Illness.* John Wiley and Sons, Inc., Hoboken, New Jersey.

Faulks S (2005). *Human Traces.* Hutchinson, The Random House Group, Ltd., London, UK.

Fink M (1999). *Electroshock: Healing Mental Illness.* Oxford: Oxford University Press.

Geller JL, Harris M (1994). *Women of the Asylum.* New York: Doubleday Anchor Books.

Gottesman II (1991). *Schizophrenia Genesis: The Origins of Madness.* New York: WH Freeman.

Gottesman II, Shields J (1982). *Schizophrenia: The Epigenetic Puzzle.* Cambridge: Cambridge University Press.

Gould SJ (1981). *The Mismeasure of Man.* New York: W.W. Norton and Company.

Henig RM (2000). *The Monk in the Garden.* New York: Houghton Mifflin.

Isaac RJ, Armat VC (2000). *Madness in the Streets : How Psychiatry and the Law Abandoned the Mentally Ill.* Treatment Advocacy Center. Toledo, Ohio: Hippo Books.

Jamison KR (1995). *An Unquiet Mind: A Memoir of Mood and Madness.* New York: Alfred A. Knopf.

Jamison KR (1999). *Night Falls Fast: Understanding Suicide.* New York: Alfred A. Knopf.

Johnstone EC, Crow TJ, Frith DC, Husband J, Krel L (1976). Cerebral ventricular size and cognitive impairment in schizophrenia. *Lancet* 2:924–926.

Kasanetz EF (1979). Tecnica per investigare il ruolo di fattori ambientale sulla genesi della schizophrenia. *Riv Psicol Anal* 10:193–202.

Kety SS, Rosenthal D, Wender PH, Schulsinger F (1968). The types and prevalences of mental illness in the biological and adoptive families of adopted schizophrenics. In Rosenthal D, Kety SS (eds.) *The Transmission of Schizophrenia.* Oxford: Pergammon, pp. 345–362.

Kingdon DG, Turkington D (2005). *Cognitive Behavioral Therapy of Schizophrenia.* New York: Guilford Press.

Kraepelin E (1907). *Etiology of Dementia Praecox, Lehrbuch Der Psychitarie,* 7th ed. Livingstone: Edinburgh.

Menninger KA (1926). Influenza and schizophrenia: An analysis of post-influenzal "dementia praecox" as of 1918 and five years later. *Am J Psychiatry* 5:469–529.

Nasar S (1998). *A Beautiful Mind.* New York: Simon and Shuster.

Nasrallah HA, Smeltzer DJ (2003). *Contemporary Diagnosis and Management of the Patients with Schizophrenia.* New York. Handbooks in Healthcare Company.

Rosenthal D (ed.) (1963). *The Genain Quadruplets: A Case Study and Theoretical Analysis of Heredity and Environment in Schizophrenia.* New York: Basic Books.

Rosenthal D, Wender PH, Kety SS, Welner J, Schulsinger F (1968). Schizophrenic's offspring reared in adoptive homes. In Rosenthal D, Kety SS (eds.) *The Transmission of Schizophrenia.* Oxford: Pergammon, 377–391.

Torrey EF (1980). *Schizophrenia and Civilization.* New York: Aronson.

Torrey EF (1984). *The Roots of Treason: Ezra Pound and the Secret of St. Elizabeths.* New York: McGraw-Hill Book Company.

Torrey EF (1988). *Nowhere to Go: The Tragic Odyssey of the Homeless Mentally Ill.* New York: Harper and Row.

Torrey EF (1998). *Out of the Shadows: Confronting America's Mental Illness Crisis*, 2nd ed. New York: John Wiley and Sons.

Torrey EF (2001). *Surviving Schizophrenia: A Family Manual,* 6th ed. New York: HarperCollins Books.

Torrey EF, Miller J (2001). *The Invisible Plague: The Rise of Mental Illness from 1750 to the Present.* New Brunswick, NJ: Rutgers University Press.

Torrey EF, Peterson MR (1976). The viral hypothesis of schizophrenia. *Schizophr Bull* 2:136–146.

Verdoux H, van Os J (2002). Psychotic symptoms in non-clinical populations and the continuum of psychosis. *Schizophr Res* 54:59–65.

A

Affect: The combination of body language, facial expression, and reactivity that signals an individual's engagement and awareness of the world around him or her.

Alzheimer's disease: One of a few progressive brain diseases that has been diagnosed in older people who appear disoriented and having difficulty communicating properly to others. A person with Alzheimer's disease has trouble remembering what happened 1 minute ago and has difficulty forming sentences and speaking, eventually progressing into not being able to take care of one's basic needs.

Amphetamines: A category of drugs that sometimes are used illicitly under names such as "speed" or "ecstasy"; they tend to produce heightened arousal and are widely abused.

Antipsychotic: Any medication that specifically suppresses the positive symptoms of hallucinations and delusions. This medication can also be useful in other conditions as a strong tranquilizer.

Attention deficit hyperactivity disorder (ADHD): A neurological disorder characterized by inattentiveness and inability to focus.

Auditory: Something that is experienced through hearing. Some schizophrenia patients have hallucinations consisting of voices speaking to them, known as auditory hallucinations.

B

Bipolar affective disorder: A psychiatric condition characterized by mood swings that occur episodically. Sometimes, particularly when very "high" (manic), people with bipolar disorder can have many of the characteristic positive symptoms of schizophrenia.

Benzodiazepines: A class of medications used in the treatment of various psychiatric disorders.

C

Cannabis: The herbaceous plant *Cannabis sativa*, the leaves of which are often smoked or ingested to produce euphoria and relaxation. The more commonly used name for this drug is marijuana. Use of cannabis has been linked with the onset of schizophrenia in at-risk individuals, and to poorer prognosis in people who continue to use it after being diagnosed with schizophrenia. Some compounds in the plant have also been developed into medications for a variety of ailments that have yet to be tested in treatment trials.

Catatonia: A condition that is characterized by extremes in behavior, of which the individual appears to be unaware. These behaviors include being mute or in a stupor and immobile to at the other extreme, being in an excitatory state of an extreme frenzy or agitated excitement. This condition is not specific to schizophrenia; although when it is periodically present in someone who has other characteristics of schizophrenia, it is then diagnosed as the subtype called "catatonic schizophrenia."

Catatonic subtype: A subtype of schizophrenia in which motor and speech changes are most prominent.

Chromosome: A structure present in the nucleus of every cell of the body of any living thing containing genes. It is shaped like a long cylinder separated into two arms that are held together in the approximate middle by a structure called the centromere. The two arms have been named "p" and "q" arms, and the length of the cylinder has been quantified by the distance from the distal tip of the "p" arm to the distal tip of the "q" arm. The "p" arm is usually the shorter of the two chromosome arms. The total distance of one chromosome is measured in "centimorgans," named after the scientist who worked out the method for measuring it, Morgan. In addition, people who view chromosomes under the microscope have noticed differences in the dark and light constitutions of the chromosome that may mean breaks in where clusters of genes start and end. Thus, a method was developed for counting these bands. The band numbers begin from the centromere and go distally using consecutively higher numbers on each arm. These two methods of measuring chromosomes and their size then gives geneticists the ability to know where different genes are located on the chromosome. Thus, when a gene is located on chromosome 6q21, 150 cM from pter, this means it is on the sixth chromosome on the longer arm (the q arm) and within the 21st band down that arm. Its exact distance from the distal tip of the p arm is 150 centimorgans. More and more information given to the public will now talk in these terms, for example: "A gene for XX disease has been found by researchers on chromosome 6q21."

Circumstantial: Wandering speech that eventually returns to its original subject.

Cognition: The quality of the mind that allows animals to think, reason, and manipulate one's environment to survive. Cognition can be measured by psychological tests. Of course, the tests are much simpler for nonhuman animals and are most complicated for humans. The well-known IQ is one measure of human cognition.

Cognitive behavioral therapy (CBT): This is a brief form of psychotherapy based on the principle that the way one thinks about something causes actions. Thus, it is focused on changing thinking patterns that lead to disruptive behavior. Several different techniques are available for CBT. This form of therapy is used for a variety of psychiatric disorders. Unlike the way it sounds, this is not a type of therapy that trains people to improve their cognition or intellectual abilities.

Command hallucinations: Imaginary voices that tell the hearer what to do.

Computed tomography (CT): A form of X-ray that is able to view the brain in more detail than a standard skull X-ray. However, it has been largely replaced by MRI as a diagnostic technique to examine details of the brain. The advantage CT has over MRI is that it detects bone change, whereas MRI views the brain tissue, and is not sensitive to bone.

Copy number variations (CNVs): Microduplications or -deletions within genes that alter gene function.

Cortex (cerebral cortex): The outer portion of the brain. It consists mostly of the "gray matter" that contains nerve cells.

D

Decompensate: To deteriorate into a less functional state.

Delusion: A false believe based on faulty judgment about one's environment.

Depression: A major psychiatric condition characterized by profound sadness all day. It is usually accompanied by physical symptoms, such as loss of appetite, loss of sleep, and slowness in movements and speech. If the condition continues as long as 1 week without relief and interferes with a person's ability to function, it is then called major depression.

Disorganized speech: Speech that is difficult to follow because topics and phrases change unexpectedly.

Dizygotic Twins: two children developing in the womb at the same time but the result of two different fertilized eggs that become implanted at the same time. These twins share DNA on average about 50 percent of time, similar to other siblings not born at the same time.

DNA: DNA is made of different nucleic acids: adenine, guanine, thiamine, and cytosine and is put together in the form of a triple helical structure. The variation in genes between individuals depends on the sequence that these nucleic acids appear in an individual's genes. DNA makes up the reproducing portion (i.e., genes) of chromosomes in animals and plants and makes up many viruses.

Dopamine: A neurotransmitter substance that is important for conveying "messages" between nerve cells in the brain.

DSM-5: The diagnostic and statistical manual developed by leading clinical psychiatrists in the United States for the systematic evaluation of psychiatric patients and assigning diagnoses to groups of symptoms. There have been five major separate revisions of this code of diagnoses since its inception.

Dyskinesia: Difficulty in performing movements voluntarily. *See also* **Tardive dyskinesia**.

E

Electroconvulsive therapy (ECT): A type of treatment usually for depression that gives a series of electrical shocks to regions of the brain given in sessions that are separated by several days. The way it exerts its effects is unknown. However, it is not dangerous or painful and is accompanied by an anesthetic when administered. The only known side effect is memory loss subsequent to the treatment.

Electroencephalogram (EEG): A type of test whereby electrodes are placed on several areas of the head and recordings are made of the brain electrical activity.

Endophenotype: A trait in genetic terms that a gene is responsible for producing and makes a person more vulnerable to getting an illness. Also called **intermediate phenotype** because it is intermediate between the gene and the clinical symptoms.

Enzymes: Proteins in the body that digest other substances through biochemical reactions. They are the "tools" of metabolism.

Estrogen: A female hormone that is produced in the female organs (ovaries). It is produced in different amounts throughout the menstrual cycle and is reduced after menopause in women.

F

Fecundity: Bearing children.

Fertility: Having the normal biology that gives one the ability to bear children.

Fish oil: A common name for compounds derived from fish that contain omega-3 fatty acids. These are substances important for the building of the lining of nerves. For good functioning of the nervous system, it is important that these fatty acids are in abundance. This is a commercial product that can be bought in health food stores at various levels of purity and has been advertised as a "cure-all" for many conditions, most of which has been unsubstantiated scientifically.

Flat affect: The appearance of being without emotion.

Functional MRI (fMRI): A brain scan that shows chemical actions taking place in the brain in response to a stimulus. The stimulus could be anything, such as voluntary movement of the fingers to memorizing a set of words.

G

Gene: A functional unit of heredity that is in a fixed place in the structure of a chromosome.

Geneticists: Scientists who study the inheritance of traits in humans, animals or plants.

Glutamate: An amino acid that is a building block of proteins. It is also by itself a major neurotransmitter in the brain (i.e., transmits information from cell to cell); by stimulating the activity of the cells, it excites them into activity.

Gray matter: The brownish gray nerve tissue of the brain and spinal cord that contains the nerve cells.

Grossly disorganized behavior: Behavior characterized by multiple factors, such as lack of self-care, unkempt clothing, strange or bizarre speech, and other socially inappropriate aspects.

H

Hallucination: Experiencing something from any of the five senses that actually is not occurring in reality (e.g., hearing voices when no one is there to speak, seeing images of things that are not really there, smelling something that is not there, feeling something touch one's body when it is not actually there, or tasting something that one is not eating).

Hippocampus: This relatively small brain structure lies deep within the temporal lobe and is thought to be crucial for memory. It has been given this name because of its unusual shape.

Homo sapiens: The scientific designation for modern human beings.

Human genome: The complete catalogue of genes and genetic variation in human DNA.

I

Immunoglobulins: The proteins that help the body respond to foreign substances and infections.

Insanity: Mental malfunctioning or unsoundness of mine to produce lack of judgment and to the degree that the individual cannot determine right from wrong. The word tends to be used in a legal context rather than a medical one.

Intermediate phenotype: The trait in genetic terms that a gene is responsible for producing, whatever makes a person more vulnerable to getting an illness. For example, an intermediate phenotype for schizophrenia may be a change in the structure of the brain that in turn may put someone at risk to get schizophrenia. Also called **endophenotype**.

L

Linkage: A genetic term that signifies a relationship between two or more genes on the same chromosome that are relatively close together so that sometimes the variations in the traits each represent are inherited together in the same individual.

Lobotomy: The surgical division of one or more brain tracts. It is usually referred to as cutting a nerve that runs from the frontal lobe to the thalamus in the brain. It has been done in various ways, most often by inserting a needle above the nose in-between the eyes. This serves to disconnect nerves connecting the frontal lobe of the brain to other structures.

M

Magnetic resonance imaging (MRI): A method to examine the tissue of the brain using a magnetic field and computer system. The machine itself consists of a horizontal tube inside of a giant magnet. The patient having an MRI scan lies on his or her back and slides into the tube on a special table. After inside, the patient is scanned.

Magnetic resonance spectroscopy (MRS): A type of MRI scan that examines chemical spectras in the brain. These chemicals are those that are present in the structure of membranes or metabolic activity in nerve cells and between cells.

Mania: A state of heightened arousal characterized by excessive emotion, e.g., elation, anxiety, fear, anger, or irritability. Behavior is characterized by fast speech and thoughts, agitation, reduced need for speech, feeling "on top of the world", and sometimes performing bizarre or risky actions.

Metabolic syndrome: A collection of metabolic risk factors that includes elevated blood pressure, dyslipidemia, decreased glucose tolerance, and weight gain, especially in the abdomen. It sometimes develops as a side effect of medication use.

Microarray: This is an orderly arrangement of DNA samples to identify many genes at one time. They can contain thousands of genes on one small plate or "chip." An experiment with a single DNA chip or microarray can provide researchers information on thousands of genes simultaneously.

Monozygotic twins: Twins born at the same time who originate from the splitting of the same egg after it has been fertilized. The DNA is identical in both twins; and thus the twins are sometimes referred to as identical.

N

Negative symptoms: Those characteristics of psychiatric illness that present as withdrawn behavior, an expressionless face, a lack of initiative, a lack of interest, not saying much when talking and saying things in short sentences, lessened thoughts, and slowed movements. Sometimes these symptoms are confused with either depression or side effects of medication.

Neurodevelopmental: Happening during the growth and formation of different structures of the brain.

Neuroleptic: Any medication that when given to animals will cause catalepsy. This name then was used to label all drugs that had an effect on reducing the symptoms of schizophrenia. In the past, neuroleptics were known as the "major tranquilizers", but the latter term is rarely used.

Neuroleptic Malignant Syndrome (NMS): A severe, although rare, side effect of neuroleptic treatment. Its underlying cause is unknown. It begins with rigidity or worsening in psychiatric symptoms despite increases in medication. Some of the warning signs are fast heart beat, high fluctuating blood pressure, tremors, sweating and fever. Cessation of neuroleptic therapy is the only treatment. It is a serious medical emergency that requires immediate attention.

O

Olfactory: Something that is experienced as an odor or scent. Some schizophrenia patients have described hallucinations that are odors.

Oxytocin: A neuromodulating hormone useful in treating some schizophrenia symptoms.

P

Paranoid: The delusional belief that people or organizations are attempting to harm one.

Pharmacotherapy: Treatment with prescription medications under the supervision of a physician.

Phenothiazines: A class of antipsychotic medications developed in the mid-twentieth century that proved useful in treating schizophrenia. These medications are known as "First-generation neuroleptics" or the "conventional neuroleptics". While many of them are still useful in some cases, they have been largely replaced with the newer "second-generation" or "atyipical neuroleptics" that tend to have fewer side effects.

Phenotype: The trait that is expressed by a gene. For example, having blue eyes or brown eyes would be phenotypes.

Pneumoencephalography: An X-ray picture of the brain taken by replacement of the cerebrospinal fluid with air or gas. This was a method used to detect whether a patient had brain atrophy prior to the invention of computed tomography and magnetic resonance imaging. This method is no longer in use.

Polypharmacy: The use of combinations of drugs to address the same problem or illness.

Positive symptoms: Considered the active symptoms of hallucinations and delusions of schizophrenia.

Positron Emission Tomography (PET): This is a radiologic procedure that measures the metabolism of a radiolabeled substance that is injected into a subject's vein and one that is known to enter the brain relatively rapidly. Pictures are then taken of the brain with the regions metabolizing the injected substance "lighting-up". PET scans are valuable tools to detect early brain tumors and have been useful in Alzheimer's research. However, they are difficult and expensive to perform, requiring a cyclotron to manufacture the radiolabeled compound and are also uncomfortable for patients. Thus, they have not been popular in recent years among schizophrenia researchers.

Premorbid: The time period before any symptoms of a disorder, including subtle signs, have developed.

Prenatal: The period between conception and birth.

Prodrome: An early or premonitory symptom of a disease. If true specific prodromal symptoms are known, one can detect the illness early. These symptoms signify that the disease will be almost certain.

Psychosis: Loss of connection with reality; experiencing delusions (i.e., false beliefs), and hallucinations. Psychotic persons often exhibit bizarre and risky behavior and do not seem to be aware that they are doing anything unusual.

R

Relapse: A recurrence of overt illness in a patient who previously had been stabilized.

Residual: Having some nonspecific symptoms (usually negative symptoms), but no longer active psychotic ones.

S

Schizoaffective disorder: Having both prominent symptoms of schizophrenia and depression and/or mania that overlap with the schizophrenia-like symptoms. However they do not always coincide so that sometimes the patients has only schizophrenia-like symptoms and other times, although less so, only mania or depressive symptoms. This diagnosis is often given by doctors without considering the whole lifetime experience of illness the patient has suffered. Often if the latter is done, the patient will have a change in diagnosis to either schizophrenia or bipolar disorder.

Schizophrenia-spectrum disorder: An alternative name for patients with schizoaffective disorder who do not show the classic symptoms.

Schizotypal personality disorder: Specific traits that are considered unusual, e.g., odd speech patterns, in a person who may not have schizophrenia.

Schizophreniform disorder: Having the symptoms of schizophrenia, but in too short a period of time (less than 6 months) to be called schizophrenia.

Stigma: Literally a "mark"; something visible to others that sets an individual apart from others whether for justified or unjustified reasons. When there is a stigma attached to a person, it is generally something that others perceive as negative.

Superior temporal gyrus: A portion of the temporal lobe of the brain that has many functions related to language, including understanding it.

T

Tangential: Speech that wanders from subject to subject and does not return to the starting theme.

Tardive dyskinesia: A debilitating motor disturbance consisting of pronounced, uncontrollable motor movements of the limbs and tongue that sometimes occurred as a side effect of older antipsychotic medications.

Tranquilizer: Any drug that is used to calm or pacify an anxious and/or agitated person. Major tranquilizers are the class of drugs used for psychotic symptoms. These terms are not often used anymore. Tranquilizer Any drug that is used to calm or pacify an anxious and/or agitated person. Major tranquilizers are the class of drugs used for psychotic symptoms. These terms are not often used anymore.

U

Unitary psychosis: The hypothesis that all schizophreniform disorders are biologically the same disease expressed differently in different individuals.

V

Ventricles: As this term applies to the brain, the spaces connecting throughout the brain that provide a system for the circulation of the fluid present in the brain called cerebrospinal fluid. The ventricles in the brain consist of the lateral ventricles, third and fourth ventricles and connect to the spinal column and bathe the spinal cord.

W

White matter: Whitish brain and spinal cord tissue composed mostly of nerve fibers and its shiny protective coat called myelin.

Working memory: This is a more contemporary term for short-term memory. It is thought of as an active system for temporarily storing and manipulating information needed for conducting complex tasks, such as learning, reasoning, and comprehending things. There are two components of working memory: storage and central executive functions. The two storage systems within working memory are for temporary storage of verbal and visual information. The central executive function is thought to be a process that is very active and responsible for the selection, initiation, and termination of the processing, the storing and retrieving of memories.

Note: Page numbers followed by *f*, or *t* indicate material in figures, or tables, respectively.

A

B

C

D

H

I

J

K

L

M

N

O

P

Q

R

S